To all the women who have lost their lives to Domestic Abuse

Hear Her Roar

Successful Women Who Experienced Domestic Abuse

The Art of Grace
PUBLISHING HOUSE

ISBN: 978-0-6452415-7-0

DISCLAIMER

The publisher takes no legal responsibility for the details inside the stories of this book. The words and opinions are the writer's own, the memories they describe are their lived experience and I do not have any evidence that those stories are untrue. I've chosen to trust the authors and have not done them the disservice of fact-checking every version of events. Memoirs are stories from one person's vantage point and these experiences are unfortunately, universal and this is why we've chosen to share them in this collection.

Although the publisher and the authors have made every effort to ensure that the information in this book was correct at press time and while this publication is designed to provide accurate information in regard to the subject matter covered, the publisher and the authors assume no responsibility for errors, inaccuracies, omissions, or any other inconsistencies herein and hereby disclaim any liability to any party for any loss, damage, or disruption caused by errors or omissions, whether such errors or omissions result from negligence, accident, or any other cause.

Some names have been changed in some stories to protect privacy.

CONTENTS

HEAR HER ROAR FOREWORD

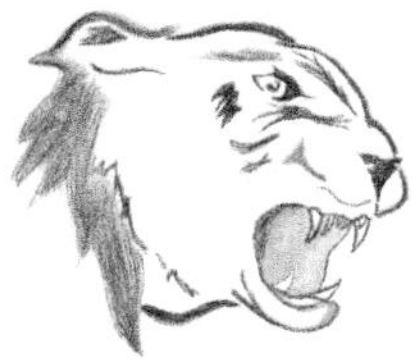

Domestic abuse is where one person uses behaviour to control another. It can involve physical violence or emotional and financial manipulation.

As a child, I was exposed to and witnessed domestic violence. Today, it makes me feel physically ill and heartsick to see that not much has changed in the world. It feels like the abuse has gotten worse, instead of better. I have a quote next to my bathroom mirror; "One person can make a difference and everyone should try" John F Kennedy. What I can do, to make a difference, even though I am only one person, is create this collaboration and talk about domestic abuse and share resources.

Since I am a publisher by trade, and story-sharing is my calling, I do what I know well: Create a place where women can share their experiences. But this book is different from any other I've put out into the world previously. It's at times darker, scarier, and even dangerous. It sheds light on a life-or-death issue that plagues our culture and that most people don't want to know about.

Here I give you 14 incredibly strong women who experienced domestic abuse and their stories and ways forward. This is our way of coming together of working toward a solution to eliminate domestic abuse and family violence.

It is heart breaking and it shocked me how incredibly easy it was to find women who shared such similar trauma. It scares me even more that I had 22 other women who were too afraid to publish their stories because they worried; "He will find me."

These words might break your heart open, make you sad and feel frustrated- well good! Use those feelings and help us do something. Anything! At the back of this book I'll provide some of the ways to seek help and give you some options and ways to seek help. If you do not feel comfortable with that, reach out to me, to one of the authors, to a friend, to someone – just do not suffer in silence.

And if you have never been in a domestic abuse situation, I would be glad if you take just one thing away let it be this- she can't "just leave", it's far more complex and nuanced than that.

THE SYSTEM

The system is fraught with bias and support to the perpetrator instead of support to the one suffering, often in silence, for fear of their or their children's lives.

SOCIETY

We need to start ostracizing the perpetrator and not the woman suffering under his control.

And we need to understand that what happens behind closed doors is very different from what we see in the streets or on social media.

Sure, it's difficult to believe that your friendly neighbor hits his wife or that your friend controls 100% of the finances in his household but these things happen. We need to trust those who are traumatized more and realise it's not easy for them to pick up and leave, especially without a plan, a lot of help and support.

SHAME

Women are not responsible for the way another person behaves. End of story.

So much shame exists around being in a domestic abuse situation or relationship. Society tends to put at least some blame upon the sufferer and you can bet they are also blaming themselves.

Perpetrators can manipulate slowly over time and coersive control is sneaky and one can not see it coming. Even if they do see it coming - they are trapped in a cycle of violence, grooming and 'love bombing.' The women easily lose their bearings.

We need to remove the shame. The only way to do that is to shed light upon it.

So here we are at the start of this book. And to you, the reader who has never experienced this, what we ask of you:

- First, please listen.
- Then use empathy to understand.
- Next, take action.

For you the woman who is planning to, desires to or is trying to leave a domestic abuse situation, we ask of you:

- Believe what is possible.
- Ask for and seek help.
- Take all the support offered.
- Leave for the children.

1

JEN SIMMS

THE FIRE

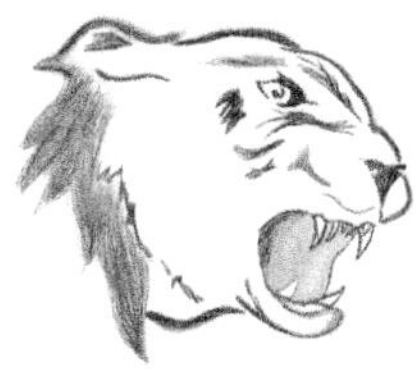

It was a Sunday morning in the Fall. That quiet sleepy Sunday was suddenly interrupted by the ringing of the phone. I remember thinking to myself, who the heck could this be calling so early? I picked up the line and answered with a polite hello. The voice on the end of the line abruptly blurts out, "there was a fire last night at the office! Someone broke in, they torched the place!" As I stood there those words washed over me, travelling from my mind, down my body into my gut. It felt as though I had received a sucker punch. I couldn't speak. That statement spun my entire world upside down. I had to go see it for myself. I don't remember the drive to get there. I can, however, recall getting out of my car, the first thing that I saw was my desk chair. I had left it tucked nicely under my desk that Friday when I left the office. There it was now lying in the grass, chard. Stepping over the yellow tape that surrounded the building I explored the scene further. Standing in the midst of the destruction, I could sense it as if he were standing there along side me. He had made good on his threats.

The fire that burned that night was a direct result, a consequence if you will, of the spark that had been lit deeply inside of me. How so? I can say with the utmost certainty that it was Divine intervention. God, Universe, Source, the power of creation itself gave me a hit on the head...literally. Nearly one year prior to that fateful night.

It is a day I will never forget. That particular day started out like any other, I had been in the kitchen preparing dinner for my husband, my daughter and myself. My youngest child had gone on an outing. My husband sat out on the front porch taking in the fall air. I popped my head out of the front door telling him dinner was done and the table set, he replied with something along the lines of he would be in shortly. As I sat at the table with my daughter, waiting and watching the minutes pass by on the clock, I began to hear voices coming from outside, they were speaking inaudibly. I decided to inquire. I got up from the table and made my way to the front porch once again. After stepping outside, I saw a man, whom I did not know standing in my front yard. The exchange of words that had begun between the two of them now escalated into arguing. My husband yelled at me, "Go back inside!"

Instead, I approached the two of them, thinking I could somehow diffuse the argument. I attempted to speak to the stranger, this I believe is what set my husband off. He grabbed the heavy wooden walking staff that had been propped up near the door and swung it. From the corner of my eye, I saw it coming. Somehow, quite miraculously, I was able to quickly step to the side, in doing so, the blow which connected with the side of my head was received with only a fraction of the force exerted behind the swing. My guardian angels were with me that night. I heard my daughter let out a frightful scream. Unbeknownst to me , she had been watching from the window. The scene broke into sheer chaos. I stumbled back to the porch and yelled out for my daughter, "Call the police!"

He continued to swing the staff. This time striking the stranger, repeatedly. I began to scream out, "STOP IT, STOP IT, you're going to kill him!!!" Then suddenly he snapped out of his rage. He threw the staff into the nearby bushes and sat down. The look on his face was as though he didn't know what had happened. The man lay motionless in the yard. The ambulance was the first to arrive, carrying the man away on a stretcher. The police came eons after and left apathetically. All in a day's work for them. I refused medical care and told the police the stranger had started the fight. It wasn't exactly a lie, it all started when he mistakenly stepped into my property.

After they left, I sat there on the front stoop in a daze. Suddenly I began to experience what I would describe as an out of body experience. I was outside of myself, hovering above, looking down upon myself sitting there, my head pulsating with pain. It was at that very moment a spark inside of me ignited. I gathered my children and checked into a hotel that night. I laid there awake, with my make-shift ice pack, quite positive I had a concussion. As I fought the urge to drift asleep, the violence of that event played out repeatedly, over and over in my mind's eye. I prayed fervently, asking God for guidance. Could I really do it? Could I leave my marriage? I was terrified.

The next day I went back home. It had taken years to get to that point. It was far easier to rationalize it all away than it was to face the reality of my circumstances. However, I was no longer in denial. I could no longer justify it. The abuse started out in the form of coercive control. A pattern of behaviors that would erode my autonomy and my self-esteem. There was a constant cycle of idealize, devalue, idealize, devalue, rinse and repeat. The idealization came mostly in the form of sweetly spoken words, followed by the devaluation, often in the form of humiliation, or acts of intimidation. Behaviors he used to gain control and power. These types of behavior are most often the precursor of physical violence. There were those instances throughout the marriage, as well. It was roughly 60 days after that incident in the front yard, that without much of a plan, I moved out of the house. The home that I had worked hard to purchase on my own merit prior to getting married, I left it. With hardly anything but my determination. I had made the decision to take my life as I knew it and burn it to the ground. Ashes to ashes, dust to dust. I thought that was the hard part. The hardest part was yet to come.

That decision was only the start of my journey and let me tell you the journey has been a long one. After all, how do you make sense of something that is completely senseless? Since the day I left, I have endured the senseless acts of a man fixated on power and control. That ultimately lead him on a path of rage and revenge. What followed for me has been an ongoing saga. The totality of consequents for me has been many. There has been a legal nightmare. There have been many, many nights of actual nightmares. There have been feelings of dread and uncertainty. It was after leaving that he began stalking, harassing and threatening me on a daily basis. This set off inside of me crippling anxiety and panic attacks. In addition to depression, anger, hopelessness, and a deep emptiness that I could not shake. My physical health began to quickly deteriorate. All of this lead me through a crash course education on the inadequacies of the American healthcare system, and its tragically flawed judicial system. Not to mention the effects this all had on my children and my relationships with them. Which has been by far the most painful part of it all.

It is my belief he thought that if he could take away my ability to support myself, I would have no choice but to come back to him. That plan failed. He began to poison the mind of the child we share. Telling sorted stories of an imaginary affair I had, in addition to a plethora of lies. Throughout the legal investigation into the fire, it was he who accused me. Claiming it was all a witch hunt. His defence was, it was me who was after him. He claimed I was trying to set him up. He claimed I had hatched a plot to get him out of the way and make off with my fictitious lover and his assets. He claimed he was innocent and to this day he has never admitted to any criminal acts and denies there was ever any form of domestic abuse on his part, in the home. There was zero logic in his so-called defence. Pointedly, it was months prior to that fire at my office, that my attorney had sent him the divorce papers stating that I wanted NOTHING from him. Not the house. MY HOUSE! Not a single cent of his money. NOTHING! All I wanted was to no longer be his wife and sole physical custody of our child. Ultimately, he was charged with five felony counts one of which was arson. However, there would be no justice. He was released from jail six months after his arrest. His charges were dismissed, due to an error made by the prosecuting attorney's office. The case was then sealed by the courts. The only remnants that there was ever a court case are the stacks of paperwork accumulated by my attorney.

The stress of it all was catching up to me. I was having nightmares regularly. I was experiencing chronic pain in my body, the origins of which were a mystery. The panic attacks were worsening to the point it felt as though I was dying. I was looking over my shoulder every second of every day. I had obtained a protection order from the court, yet he continued to stalk me. I filed countless reports to the police to no avail. It became insurmountable, I started to have suicidal thoughts. I felt hopeless. I couldn't see a way out even though I had left him. I sought help for myself by making an appointment with my doctor. I shared everything through streams of tears. I did not receive much in the way of understanding from my male physician. Through no fault of his own, they don't exactly teach how to handle these situations in medical schools. There was no referral to services for domestic abuse survivors. There were no statistics shared on the prevalence of domestic violence. I was told to "manage my stress." I was referred to a psychiatrist. I was handed written prescriptions for a cocktail of anti-anxiety and anti-depressant medications. I felt labelled. I felt completely alone. I did not go there in search of better living through pharmacology. When I left that doctor's office, I knew that it was up to me and me alone to save myself. I decided right then and there. I was done with suffering. It was completely unsustainable. I decided to take a hard look in the mirror. I needed to understand how I got to this place in life. I sat in all the feelings, the shame, the guilt, the self-judgement, the self-destructive tendencies. I knew I was better than that. I decided to become the heroine of my story.

I began to let all of the broken pieces of myself fall away. I forgave it all. And I set out to educate myself, searching out every book I could find on the topics of personality disorders. Reading up on narcissists, psychopaths, sociopaths, cluster B's, I studied them all. I was damn determined to make some sort of sense of it all. What I learned was that the man I married, perfectly mirrored back to me all of my brokenness. He is essentially identical to my father. The same heavily masculine toxic energy. My father was an abuser. I am the product of a domestic abuse household. I never talked about it to anyone. It was a dirty little secret. My mother suffered at his hands for years. The abuse spilled over into the relationships with my siblings. My mother's children from her first marriage. I was always thankful I shared his DNA as I felt this is what spared me from that sort of treatment. I felt guilty at times. I carried around my father's sins in secret. I spent so many years burying the pain from my so-called childhood, that I inadvertently buried my intuition right along with it. Lacking self-awareness, I attracted the very same "type" of man. Rest in peace Dad. I love you and I forgive you.

After reading volumes and volumes of books, I concluded that I had married the King of the narcissist. For those of you unfamiliar with this term let me define it. A narcissist is a person with a grandiose admiration and opinion of themselves. They are completely devoid of empathy. They intentionally cause harm to others without any sense of remorse or responsibility. They pray on forgiveness. They manipulate compassion and exploit sympathy. They will wage warfare against you literally and psychologically leaving you feeling humiliated and shameful. This is exactly how they want you to feel. I used to justify his behavior by telling myself love endures all things. Isn't that what they say? Love endures all things. Only it wasn't love. It was conditioning.

In addition to educating myself. I had to do the inner work. It took going back, way back into my timeline and healing my wounded inner child. Giving her all the love, attention, affirmation and respect, she needed and never got. In addition, I found an amazing online support group for survivors. I started to go for long runs in nature. I did a green juice cleanse. I started meditating. I journaled. I continued to pray. I started to love and honor myself each day. It took some time but I did it. Just as my former husband eroded my humanness piece by piece. Each new day I took my power back, piece by piece. And guess what? I healed myself. Physically. Mentally. Emotionally. Spiritually. I have broken old patterns and cycles. And I have created new, healthy ones. I have developed my intuition. In the end, I'm grateful for all of the tribulation. It has taught me a great deal about myself and my strengths. I came out of it knowing who I am truly meant to be.

It was in the midst of my healing journey that I became re-acquainted with the gift that I had known innately as a child, I always had. I am a true empath. Acknowledging this was the start of my experimenting with energy healing modalities. Ultimately leading me to become a certified crystal healer. After this I studied Dr. Mikao Usui which led me to become a Reiki Master, I then went on to become an accredited meditation teacher. Through my own journey, I developed a powerful methodology for holistic healing. I then felt the call to share my methods with other women, in 2018 I founded Zen by Jen Holistic Healing. I have had the great honor to work with women from all around the globe, assisting them on their own unique path to healing, utilizing my tried-and-true methodology.

The woman sitting here today is a vastly different woman than she once was. Although the saga continues for me, due to the fact I share a child with my abuser and now a grandchild. I have many things to be grateful for. Each new day I walk further down the path of my purpose. The best is yet to come. I'm excited for every new person that I meet and every new opportunity that knocks at my door. I rose out of the depths of hell and I opted for forgiveness. I proudly carry the scars of yesterday, they are a reminder of the lessons turned to wisdom. They are a reminder of how I turned humiliation into triumph and how I learned to surrender to the power of my soul. Ultimately, it was all a lesson, not a life sentence.

My story is just one. There are many women like me. Statistics from the National Coalition Against Domestic Violence state that on average 1 in 7 women have experienced abuse by their domestic partner. 1 in 10 are raped by their partner. Tragically there is mounting data that suggest these numbers have shot up worldwide since the beginning of the pandemic with the lookdowns that have followed. On a typical day, there are 20,000 calls made to domestic violence hotlines. It has become a crisis within the crisis. If you need assistance please reach out. The National Domestic Violence Hotline is free and available 24/7 at 1-800-799-SAFE or text the word START to 88788 or visit www.NCADV.org Abusers often look through search history and call logs, take precautions to delete any information from your phone or computer that may tip someone off.

Remember dear one,
You are LOVE
You are Light
You are a Soul
You are Brave
You are Strong
You are Unique
You are Special
And no matter what is happening in your life...YOU GOT THIS!
Together we RISE.

JEN SIMMS

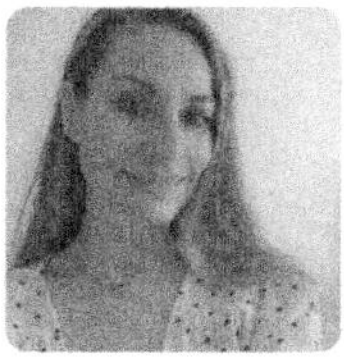

Jen Simms is the founder of Zen by Jen Healing. She utilizes energy medicine within her powerful three-fold methodology, facilitating natural healing for women in search of a holistic path to releasing and healing trauma.

Jen specializes in assisting women with emotional recovery after abuse. Originally, Jen worked within her local community to advocate for women. In 2020, she began to expand her reach by working virtually with women from around the world.

Jen Simms is a Certified Reiki Master, Certified Crystal Healing Practitioner, Certified Meditation Teacher, Author, Speaker, and Women's Advocate.

Contact Jen...
Website: www.ZenbyJenHealing.com
Facebook: www.facebook.com/ZenbyJenHealing
Email: Jen@ZenbyJenHealing.com

2

KIZIAH JAY

BREAKING SILENCE

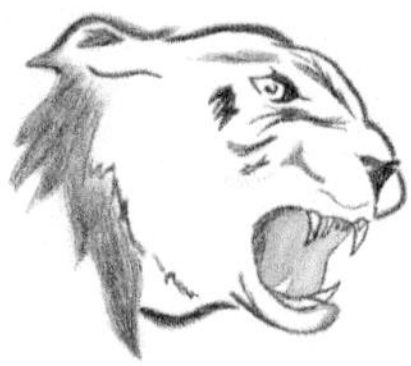

She was the most beautiful woman I had ever seen. As I sat there quietly taking in her beauty, I noticed the blanket she was knitting my baby brother draped over her bump.

At around 6 years old my mummy was my whole world.

I loved my daddy too. He was big and strong, and he loved plants. There was something else, something which made me scared, scared of him.

Sometimes he would get very mad and hurt my mum. Sometimes he would upend the dinner table with our meals mummy had made for us and food would go everywhere. Plates smashed, crying, screaming. Then mummy would send us to our rooms to play so she could clean up the mess.

As I sat and watched her create this beautiful blanket for her unborn baby, my brother, I became aware of noise around me as my sister ushered me into our bedroom. With our bodies pressed against the door and hands over our ears , we stared at one another terrified.

Mummy was crying and begging him to stop. She was yelling "the baby!".

In those moments I wanted to open the door and help my mummy, but I was too little. I was also scared.

When she woke us up in the middle of the night and told us we were going on a holiday. I didn't question it. I felt safe with her and knew I would be okay.

We moved to a small remote town and that would be our lives for the next three years. We never went back to our home, we walked away with the clothes on our back and started our new lives.

I never asked where my dad was.

A few years had passed, and we made another move, this time to Sydney NSW. Mum was happy, we were all adjusted and got to see our cousins regularly. Life was good.

I came home from school one day and there was a strange man in our house. He was on the lounge talking with my mum. She beamed "hello Kiz, meet my friend"

Less than a week later this man was living in our house, and sleeping in my mum's bed, and I was not happy. There was something about him I didn't like but Mum seemed happy, so I kept my feelings about him to myself.

It wasn't long before I started to notice Mum behaving strangely.

Walking home one day, it was about 40 degrees outside, and I was so thirsty. I picked up my pace so I could get home faster. I opened the front door and walked inside. As I got closer to the kitchen I turned to the hallway on my left.

There she was, unconscious, levitated off the ground by the neck with his one strong arm. His face looked unrecognizable to me, his eyes glazed over and veins popping from his neck. In those moments I froze.

I jumped as I heard him scream for me to help him, "chuck her in the bath". He ran the cold shower over her, and I watched in horror as he slapped her face and body to try and wake her.

We moved her to the bed and as I lay beside her lifeless body, he whispered in my ear... "She will never leave me, I have her wrapped around my little finger."

My heart was beating faster and faster. I didn't show him I was afraid. I didn't show any emotion. I didn't want him to see.

As a young woman finding her feet in the world this made an impact on me that shook the life from me for a long time.

A light went out in my mum that day and to this day I haven't seen it come back on.

While it went out for her it came on for me. I had to be the strong one. I was the eldest now, I had to do something, I had to protect her.

It wasn't long before I realized what I was up against. The more life spiraled out of control at home. the angrier I got.

Mum wouldn't listen to me, and he would threaten or hurt mum to keep me submissive and keep my mouth shut.

Tell her to shut her mouth or you will cop it again. She would beg me to keep quiet, but I didn't want him to think he could do this to us. Every time I spoke, he would send her flying to the ground with another punch, kick, hit or push.

That day I lost my own voice.

I learnt to be silent, so as not to cause him to go off.

We soon learnt he was a heroin addict and had been in and out of prison his whole life.

It didn't matter, it was too late. My mother married him.

My childhood felt like being on a rollercoaster with no option to get off and feel safe.

I lived in a constant state of fear which affected every aspect of my life.

Often lying to my friends when I was asked to come to their place so I could stay home and watch my mother.

It was around this time she began to overdose and cut her wrists.

There were periods where I would need to call the ambulance almost every day to take her to the hospital.

Most of the time this happened when my stepfather was due to be released from jail.

Even so, it wasn't uncommon to spend every weekend at the prison courtyard so mum could see him.

Over time, I didn't mind it and found myself falling for a 20 something year old inmate and we became pen pals. It turned out he was in there for rape.

I suppose it kept me occupied and I loved the attention I got. So, it didn't take much coercing when mum told us we would be spending Christmas day at the prison. I still have the family photo of us all with Santa hats on and smiling.

I never believed any of my childhood to be anything but normal.

Driving around the streets at night with us all piled in the car on school nights was an adventure, sometimes I would even invite my closest friend for the ride!

Women's shelters weren't so bad either. I met a boy my age there one time. He looked like a young Kurt Cobain. We comforted each other and made things fun.

The thing about that was that he always seemed to find a way to find us, then we would have to find another shelter which sucked especially after I had made some friends.

It didn't matter anyway; she would always take him back and the cycle would repeat over and over.

I didn't think we would ever get away from him. He would threaten to take us all up into the mountains and bury us alive if Mum tried to leave him.

The police didn't do much about the threats, even though they knew him they couldn't do much until he had done something. Even then it would be just an overnight stay in the cells before he was released to come and stalk and harass us again until Mum would give in and bring him back into our home.

She managed to put him in prison twice after beating her up, but even then, we weren't safe.

Mum had always been an early riser and so by the time we awoke she would have normally drawn open the curtains to let light in. This morning however as I walked out of my room to the bathroom, I noticed the house was dark and I couldn't hear anyone awake.

As I thought this was a bit odd, I just assumed Mum was still asleep and must have been very tired.

When I got to the bathroom door it was closed and I noticed my stomach begin to churn as I could hear her soft whimpers. The door opened and there she was, sitting in the bath naked, head between her legs sobbing.

I repeatedly asked her what was wrong and to look at me. She slowly pulled her face away from her body and my heart sank.

The bruises and black eyes told me everything I needed to know. All she said was rape.

I don't know what happened next, but I do know I was furious. Livid. Heartbroken.

What Mum didn't know at the time was that I used to read her diary. This had begun about a year earlier when she would start hiding things from me. I needed to know what was going on. If she wasn't going to do something I was.

It was around 6 weeks before this incident that I read Mum had been receiving threatening calls, vividly explaining what was to happen to her. It included coming into her home, bashing, and raping her. I honestly don't know how she kept this to herself. She must have been so frightened.

It turns out, as we three kids slept that night, my stepfather organized a drug addict friend of his to come to our house, break-in and bash and rape her in her own bed.

The reason was so he could tell the court that he needed to be released earlier to come home and look after his wife and kids as they were in danger.

I guess to make it more believable he thought he would up the ante in the form of getting someone to come around one morning. as I tied my shoelaces before leaving for school one morning on the lounge right in front of a window I was horrified as a massive concrete boulder flew right past my head shattering and smashing the glass which fell all over me.

Did his games work? Yes. He was released soon after and the cycle began again.

I found myself becoming increasingly angry at life and I started to dabble in recreational drugs and alcohol.

I would fantasize about a different life. The one I thought about most was having a home, that felt safe. One we didn't need to run from. One that didn't hold bad memories. And one that was full of smiles, laughter, and love. I had a great imagination and used this vividly to escape my reality at home.

I seemed to have adopted a few new habits and behaviors which helped me escape my troubled mind.

By 16 restricted my diet so that I was only eating every few days and even then, it would be something usually with a high dose of sugar to keep me going. I was on medication for depression and taking on risky behavior.

The more dangerous the better. Anything which gave me a rush would excite the hell out of me.

Sneaking out of home at night was one.

A good friend of mine, at the time, and I wagged school that one day. We ran into three guys who were about 19-20 years old. She seemed to know them so when they invited us around that night I wasn't fazed.

Even if I was, I feel like I wouldn't have said anything. People-pleasing became something I had also adopted in any attempt to receive love from others.

So that night I went to her house, and we waited until 11pm when her parents were asleep and snuck out to walk about two kilometers to this guy's house.

It was cold, wet and raining. We were dressed in summer clothing and as we walked through tall grass and bush, I started to regret our decision.

Still,. I didn't say anything and as we finally reached their house and opened the door, we were both asked if we would like a drink.

My friend said yes to an alcoholic drink, but I said no and was given a bottle of coke instead.

There was something about these guys that made me feel uncomfortable, but I felt safe with my friend and as she chatted away to them, I sat silent pretending to engage in the conversation.

The next thing I remember is being passed over a fence. I was in and out of consciousness and could hear male voices.

The next thing I remember is trying to open my eyes and noticing I was under a tree, the grass felt wet beneath me, and someone was having sex with me. I could hardly see or move, and I remember feeling like I wanted to cry and scream but I couldn't. There was another male there and I heard him say hurry up, my turn next.

I must have blacked out again and I woke up to a male sitting over me with a torch between my legs laughing about the hole they had made in my underwear. I could hear other people laughing.

I started to freak out wondering where I was and where my friend was when I heard her voice. She was laughing with them.

At some point, I had tried to stand up and I was all over the place, I was sobbing, my heart was beating out of my chest and my stomach was in pain because my bladder was so full.

I told her that I wanted to go home but she brushed me off and told me to just wait until morning.

I was horrified. I felt scared and alone.

The rest of the night is wiped from my conscious awareness however my unconscious mind seemed to remember everything because the following weekend as we met my stepfather in the prison courtyard for his two-hour visit, my mother handed him a piece of paper.

Apparently, she had found a detailed two-page letter I had written explaining everything.

I felt so humiliated. I was angrier than ever, and I chose not to charge them.

My self-worth started to take a nosedive, I became withdrawn and started to sleep a lot. When I was not out drinking myself into a stupor, I was taking anything, I could get my hand on.

The good news is we finally got away from my mum's partner and moved interstate.

At 19 after a bad break-up, no job or money, I found myself walking into a brothel and signing up for what would be my first shift of many.

Some would say it would be self-explanatory what to do but I was horrified when the madam just gave me a quick tour and showed me to the girl's room out the back.

Talk about being thrown in the deep end!

I soon learnt my first client was a regular they frequently called to take the new girl to see how she went and if she could handle it.

Apparently, I passed because that became my home for the next almost four years.

The girls became my family and looked after me like a little sister and I loved them.

Life in those four years and how I exited is for another story, another chapter, perhaps another book.

What I do know for certain is that throughout my whole life I intuitively knew somehow and somewhere I would use my story to help others and this thought brought me through many times where I wanted to give up.

In 2017, in my third year of a nursing degree, I hit rock bottom.

I found myself carefully planning exactly how I would end my life one night while my children slept.

It would be the same way my father committed suicide.

As I said goodnight to them that night I gave them extra time, extra hugs, and extra love.

I had made my decision, there would be no coming back.

Seconds before I took the action that would end my life, I felt a sudden overwhelming sense of comfort and love envelope me and I sat still in time, the only sounds of my own sobs.

After this, something changed in me.

Every single day, sometimes every single moment, I chose life. No matter the cost.

Not too long after, and in perfect timing I was led on a journey of self-discovery and healing. What I had discovered for myself was so profound and powerful that I became an NLP coach so that I can help support other women in taking back their power.

It takes an incredible amount of strength, resilience, and courage to leave a Domestic Violence situation but staying steals your soul, along with your identity and dreams.

Domestic Violence from a child's perspective is a hopeless one. Watching my mothers light go out in her eyes was the most heartbreaking of all.

She is my biggest inspiration for the work that I do now in supporting women in the adult industry transition out of the industry, heal and come back home to themselves in a way that empowers them to be all of who they were born to be.

Turning my pain in to my greatest power was the catalyst for creating the life that I have and will continue to.

Every woman deserves a life and relationship which she is not afraid to be herself. One where she is free to be independent and treated and spoken to with respect. One where she is not afraid. One where she can close her eyes at night and not be in fear. One where she does not question herself because of the doubt put in her mind.

Every woman deserves to know and feel in every cell of her being that she matters, that she is worthy and that she is irreplaceable.

We all have a past; we all have a story. When we speak up, when we use our voice, when we are heard we give others permission to do the same.

We were not born to live in shame, insignificance, and unworthiness. That is not our story. It's not your story. We are survivors. You are a survivor.

I believe in you, I was you, I am you and I love you.

KIZIAH JAY

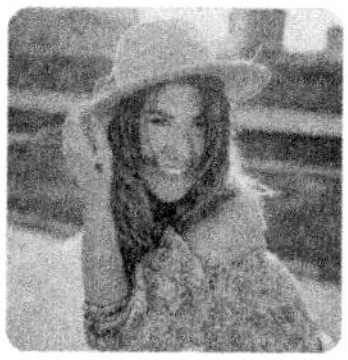

Kiziah Jay is a 41-year-old mother of 3 extraordinary kids living in Queensland, Australia.

Kiziah Jay is no stranger to adversity and has experienced considerable hardships including domestic violence, rape, traumatic childhood, a mother who repeatedly self-harmed and suffered from borderline personality disorder, her father committing suicide, eating disorders and body dysmorphia, depression and working as a prostitute for almost 4 years.

Kiziah Jay intuitively always knew she would use her experiences to impact the lives of others one day and tells how this thought gave her strength in her darkest hours.

Kiziah Jay never give up attitude has been a catalyst for her drive and success to being deeply committed to helping women who are lost in their relationships reclaim their power and identity and ultimately feel empowered.

Kiziah Jay is a passionately fierce woman who cares deeply for humanity and is creating impact on a global scale through her work.

Website: www.kiziahjay.com
Book a call with me: www.calendly.com/kirsty-37/60min
Apple Podcast: www.podcasts.apple.com/au/podcast/shes-priceless/id1593538149

3

MYRA FORDHAM

HOW I BECAME AUSTRALIA'S #1 TRAUMA COACH FOR WOMEN

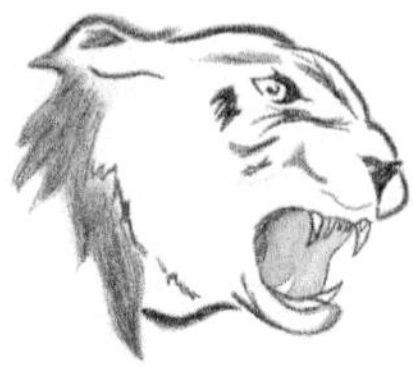

I believe the trauma that I carried was passed down to me genealogically, it started from in the womb and continued after birth throughout my life for as long as I can remember.

In my teens, my father was my best friend, the person I trusted with my life. Every time we had a disagreement he would always apologise and say that he would never hurt me and wanted me to always be happy which I know was the truth.

My father was my protector and my rock. We would always talk to each other almost every day on the phone. He was always there for me when I needed guidance or to chat and unload.

In 2015 is where I met my ex, the "new guy" on the world-famous dating app called "Tinder" just after I broke up with another ex. I shared with the new guy that I only wanted sex, company, and absolutely, no strings attached. It started with us chatting a lot on Tinder every day. I was attracted to him only because of his muscles, not his face, and because he knew a lot about the gym and cars. Plus, he was giving me the attention I craved.

I remember the first time I met him it was so awkward he hid under his baseball hat. The first time we met and slept together. As I laid on his chest and looked into his eyes and my intuition communicated to me odd feelings towards him with my gut feeling, no good. I verbally affirmed that " There's something about you, I just don't know what it is about you, I am not sure if it's good or bad but I will find out later" I continued because his mysterious behaviour intrigued me.

I shared my intentions with him that I only wanted fun and nothing serious. Because I just left a toxic relationship, the guy I was with before left me for a friend of mine, so I was healing from that.

As we continued to see each other, we spent a lot of time together. He used to spoil me with food, wined and dined, gave gifts, and trained me at the gym. He also showed me how to service cars and was a handyman. The sex was good at the start. This sounds too good to be true right?

Well, this is where I share the first red flag.

1. He was telling his workmates that I was his girlfriend. Which was untrue and incorrect information, I said that was bullsh*t!

2. He started to be extra clingy.

3. He was nice to my dog, then when she did something bad, he kicked and punched her violently. She soon became petrified of him...

I called him out on his violent behaviour.

This is when everything started to turn upside down and hundreds of red flags were raised.

4. He would touch me inappropriately in my sleep—I told him not to, because of my childhood trauma and how it made me feel unsafe.

5. Then he sexually assaulted me, choke slammed me onto the bed, and touched me while I said "No! Stop!"—I felt so sexually violated and got very upset.

He packed up his stuff and went home. This raised so many alarm bells and had me questioning myself "What the f*ck Myra, why would you allow that?"—I cried and felt so gross because of what he did to me.

I messaged him and begged him to come back, wanting him around because I was lonely and wanted to be loved.

6. I was eating food on the bed, and I pretended to cut his leg with a blunt butter knife. He then grabbed the knife and punched my thigh hard with force. This created a bruise that I kept photos of. I cried and begged for him to come back and then we both apologised to each other, and he said that he would never hurt me again. We then went shopping and he bought me a black dress, perfume and some basketball shoes for the gym.

7. He lied about his age, he looked way too old to be 28, I found his ID later and it said 32.

Even though we said sorry and made up, I still wanted to report it to the police and my family, however, I felt disempowered and lost. I then carried guilt, shame, anger, and sadness. Not knowing what to do because I would potentially lose someone who cared for me.

I later learned that he was into drugs and steroids which was a mask, he wore to be someone he was not. He showed me how to inject his shoulder with steroids. I felt pressured and just did it because I liked him.

I began to think" wow, is this normal? How weird for someone to act like this and treat someone they care about like dirt.

We decided to become official on Facebook.

He opened up to me and shared that when he was a child, he used to watch his father beat his mother. This is where I first had my "Ah-ha" moment. This is why he carried on with this type of behaviour and continued to display his childhood trauma into our relationship.

I started working away from home out at sea. It was challenging being away from a clingy man. I remember us always arguing and blaming each other for cheating. It was so immature, and both of our insecurities came out to play and caused chaos. I remember calling him every few days. He then shared that he loved me. It was weird because I didn't know how to feel or react appropriately.

I would also call my Dad often and check in to see how he was and share my new learnings and adventures.

There was one day in December 2015 where I called him to see how he was. Dad said he had a health check-up at the hospital. There he found out that he had stage 2 aggressive cancer and had 2-8 weeks to live. This news crushed my heart. It felt like a part of me was slowly dying. As I worked on deck, it was like it wasn't there in my body. I felt empty and could not concentrate. I then left the vessel and flew to Sydney to spend the last days with my father. As I arrived, I felt relieved but also like my world was ending. I saw my dad and uncle's for the first time again in months, I broke down crying because I never realised how serious my father's cancer was. He appeared to be just skin and bone. It killed me to see this, that year was the worst time of my life. I had to care for my dad because that is what family does. I was young and selfish and complained about not doing my own thing and wasn't going to the gym. How heartless of me to say! As I write this, I am crying so loud from the pain. It is releasing my trapped emotions, to heal this part of me that I have felt guilt for all these years. The one thing that I remember Dad saying was "Myra when I get better, I am going to take you on a holiday, just you and me, okay?" I replied, "Yes Dad, that would make me very happy." I then sobbed next to him in the room while I lay next to him on his bed. A couple of days later I witnessed my father die slowly, gasping for air in the hospital.

My heart was now shattered into more tiny pieces. My ex flew down to support me at my father's funeral.

Later that year, on October 24th, 2016 all I remember is having food with my ex-partner at the time and that was it.

Everything I shared with you I thought was normal up until the point that I nearly died and woke up in a hospital bed. I found out he physically abused me and then king hit me in the head while I was washing the dishes.

I now identify as having an invisible injury; a bilateral subdural hemorrhage within my temporal lobes and my right lateral temporal parenchymal contusions and subarachnoid hemorrhage. I also had a 2 mm midline shift. Following the traumatic brain injury (TBI), I had difficulties with attention, concentration, reduced verbal fluency, and difficulty following complex commands. I am still recovering to this day. I now experience cognitive impairments.

After the news from the doctors and nurses, I was shocked, sad, but also glad that he did me a favour because this ended our abusive, toxic, insecure relationship.

I learned that I was in an induced coma for 11 days.

Let me share one of life's biggest mysteries with you. When I was in a coma, I could hear and feel everything around me, people's voices, people talking to me. However, I was dreaming that I was living my life, going to work each day, and felt fully conscious. Be careful what you say around people that are in a coma because they might hear you and remember.

I then learned that I couldn't walk or talk, even though my mind knew how. It was as though my body was responding differently. In my mind I was fully capable but, my body said no. My balance was so bad. I remember having to be escorted to the bathroom and shower in a wheelchair.

This was a kick in the guts. I started to feel useless, like a baby, and my privacy and independence were robbed from me.

I used to sleep a lot and get really bad tension and headaches. I remember being woken up heaps so that I could take my morphine medication and blood thinner injection in the stomach every day. I recall the nurses supervising me while I was trying to go to the bathroom and take a shower. It was extremely uncomfortable. I recall my mother having to brush my teeth in the hospital bed. I felt like a baby, and it made me cry and feel sad and powerless. I remember being pushed in a wheelchair to attend my appointments at the rehabilitation services. I had countless therapies and rehab appointments such as, Occupational therapy, speech therapy, physiotherapy, counselling, psychology, and doctor's appointments. My license was suspended due to the severity of the Traumatic brain injury.

I had to attend numerous court hearings, involving my ex-partner which were painful. I got to see him for the first time, I saw him for who he was, just an average joe without access to steroids and skinny. He then mouthed “sorry” as I looked at him in the face. I looked at him blankly with anger and rage.

I thought to myself how the hell can someone who is meant to love and care about you, cause so much damage, trauma, and pain?

Finally, the court process ended. He only received just under four years of jail time. Which in my opinion is pathetic, this man almost killed me. He robbed me of my independence. Luckily my family was home and called the police and the paramedics... My sister said she saw everything. I do not recall anything. She said she screamed at him, he punched me directly in the head, my cranium hit the bench and my head hit the tiles on the hard floor.

He then ran into the room and gathered all his belongings and disappeared into thin air.

The one scary and most alarming thing that the police mentioned was that they found him at work carrying on living his life as if nothing had happened. That made me feel sick inside! Punching the "love of your life" in the head and almost killing her and pretending that nothing happened". They then brought him into lockup, questioned him and took him into custody until the case was solved.

I cried each night while in hospital and wanted to go home to be with my dog and her puppies. I finally was granted home visitation rights which made me happy! While in hospital, I noticed that I suffered from photophobia. This is a condition where the person is sensitive to light. They had to stick trash bags over the windows for me. I was also irritable to noise and perfumes and different scents. I moved into a single room. My carers washed my clothes and helped me a lot. I then got an early release to go home! I felt free but still not independent!

I first went to the local supermarket to buy food and toiletries. I soon discovered that I had severe social anxiety and panic attacks. This was a shock to the system because I genuinely thought I was good. I noticed that I was shaking, my breath was quick, I was looking around panicking paranoid, and thinking that everyone was staring at me judging me. It was hell! However, I know now this was just my perception.

I found it hard to sleep because I was sensitive to every noise. I experienced mood swings of pure anger, frustration, and sadness. I could not control my emotions. I fell into the deepest darkest hole in depression and experiencing anxiety. I started to have suicidal thoughts to end all the pain, to be with my father in heaven.

I would cry often and want to break things violently. The only thing that kept me happy was my dog and her pups. I also had to avoid screen time, being on my phone, watching movies, and playing Xbox.

I was unable to work 12-hour days like I used to. I couldn't receive a disability pension from the government. Things were tough! I then came up with an idea to create a crowdfund campaign. A friend helped me to raise funds for my occupational therapy driving assessment. I raised enough to keep me going for the time being.

My mother and sister took time off work to care for me which I am grateful for now. I can only imagine how stressful it was for them.

In December a mutual friend introduced me to her friend Sam, from the United Kingdom. It was his birthday! Sam a dry seat next to him and I happily accepted, pretending that I didn't want to. Sam was cheeky and nice. I shared with him why I couldn't drink to celebrate his birthday, (because of my TBI) so he got me water instead. I thought this was so nice. Little did I know that I met my twin flame and the man of my dreams, the love of my life. We then swapped contacts and kept in touch. We decided to meet up and go on a date. I was hesitant due to my past trauma and how another man almost killed me. So, I shared my intentions with Sam that I just wanted to have company and no relationship. Sam understood, he was kind and compassionate. Even though he didn't know me well, he treated me exactly how a woman deserves to be cared for. He bought me dinner at a fancy restaurant, dessert, and was a great host at his apartment in the city. I decided to go with the flow, however, I was guarded like the Great Wall of China. But the little girl in me wanted to be loved and accepted for who I was. The love I craved from my childhood.

Sam and I began getting to know each other more, we stayed up late chatting. I felt like a schoolgirl again, excited, playful, and happy

Christmas is now approaching December 2016! Sam invited me over for the weekend. He took me shopping. He said okay Myra your limit is $100 or you can get 2 items, $250 later I had my Christmas gifts ready from Santa.

In January 2017 I got medically cleared to go back to the gym and slowly get on my feet again.

Months later Sam and I decided to become official in a committed relationship and live together, I finally left the nest. It was one of the best things I have done in my life! Sam supported me fully with my continual recovery and he worked while I stayed at home. I ended up being cleared by the doctors to work a maximum of four hours. I struggled to keep up with the other workers so I sadly had to leave several workplaces because they could not support my needs with my cognitive impairments.

As my relationship with Sam progressed, I noticed my shadow creeping up in which I was jealous, insecure, and had trust issues. I became an "askhole" because I was unable to make complex decisions on my own. I would always ask for Sam's guidance and had to run everything past him to be certain.

I noticed myself lashing out at Sam because I never knew how to control my emotions, and old trauma and repressed emotions would resurface. There were a few times in our relationship where I felt so guilty for not being a good partner and that I would neglect him, treat him badly and call him names. I had this awakening that I had to change because it wasn't serving our relationship.

I started my life coaching qualification in 2020 and it honestly was one of the best things I invested into, my personal growth. Regardless of the price, I needed something new and exciting to help my ongoing TBI recovery. It taught me how to unlearn my victim mindset mentality, how to heal, remove negative thoughts, become a better person, and become more positive. It was the key to all my past trauma and pain!

I started to coach women to help them make some serious lifestyle changes to become the best versions of themselves to heal, forgive and surrender to love.

This journey was so challenging and tough, however, it taught me how the human subconscious mind works and why people behave in certain ways. Life coaching also taught me how to uninstall old habits and limiting beliefs that people have been holding on to since birth and how to reinstall good habits and new positive belief systems.

Life coaching has changed my outlook on life and how someone who hit rock bottom and almost got killed can change the trajectory of their lives and open a business!

I have been married to Sam for over four years and we are both in love and give to each other with no expectations.

I am now a Published Co-author in a book

I am Australia's #1 Trauma Coach for women.

What I do is help women who struggle with trauma to heal themselves and break free! My exclusive 6 week Boss Lady Breakthrough programs only run 3 times a year and are available upon application.

Here are 6 learnings/lessons I would love to share with you

1. Look out for the red flags in a relationship and odd behaviours.

2. You have the choice to walk away at any time and seek professional help.

3. Inner work is something that we just press the pause button when we are tired, angry, upset, or frustrated. Inner work is a continual cycle of life.

4. Always remember to self-love and care for yourself, fill up your love cup so then it overflows into others. Put yourself first before others so then you can give love to other people who truly need it.

5. Invest into your personal development spiritual journey, you cannot put a price on your mental health and wellbeing. You only live once, so make it a good one.

6. No matter how much inner work you have practiced or how positive you are, there's always more to do. It is a never-ending process. Healing is extremely uncomfortable, and we always store suppressed emotions and trauma below the surface so healing never stops.

MYRA FORDHAM

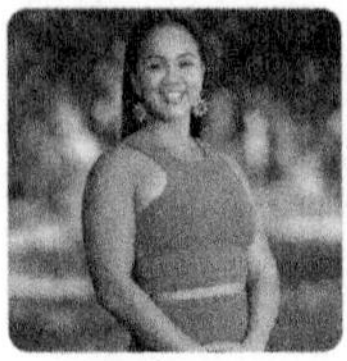

Myra Fordham is Australia's #1 Trauma Coach for Women.

She is a First Nations Malgin Gurindji, woman from Kalkaringi, Wave Hill NT, Australia.

Myra helps professional women to heal past trauma to become happy and free.

Back in October 2016, Myra was physically abused by her ex-partner. As a result, Myra was left fighting for her life and sustained an invisible Traumatic Brain Injury.

Myra was determined to heal and relearn how to walk and talk again.

Myra is a powerful heart-centered, high-energy, results-driven coach.

Ladies, give yourself the greatest gift to become happy and free with Myra's services!
If you feel spiritually called to work with Myra on a deeper level, please apply for her 6-week Boss Lady Breakthrough program and take immediate action now!
https://bit.ly/sistime

Tune in for your "Daily dose of Myra Motivation"
https://bit.ly/myrafordham

Join Myra's free tribe today!
https://bit.ly/My-Ra

4
YAMALIT HOLGUIN
YOUR PAST DOES NOT DEFINE YOU

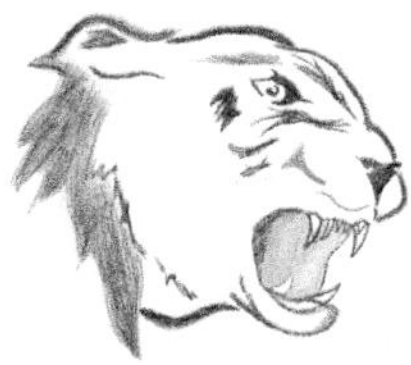

What is the hardest thing to overcome they ask? Our self-doubt would be the first thing that comes to mind. My name is Yamalit Holguin (Yami for short), a first-generation immigrant, fresh from Venezuela to good old New York. I came to New York at just three months old, my parents clearly, fearless, and ready for a fresh start. I grew up in the Bronx, up until I was 14when I moved to where I reside now, a cute little town named Beacon, NY. Let's fast forward to my first week of college, freshman year.

I had two sisters, one older, one 7 years younger, and one little brother. In my first week of college, I got a call from my older sister, Judy. She was frantic, our little sister Yumelit had been experiencing severe headaches for a few days (to the point of throwing up) and the local hospitals had brushed us off. My older sister was bringing Yumelit down to NY Presbyterian in Manhattan, and asked if I wanted to come. "Of course," I said. I packed some clothes and waited to be picked up.

At the hospital, they took her in immediately, they took her straight for an MRI. It seemed like an eternity before she was back. An even longer eternity while we waited for the results. My sister, my mother and I, all guessing on what it could be. The nurses and Doctor walk in and pull us away from my baby sister. One nurse is crying, while the Doctor stuttered to explain what they had found; a tumor in the middle of her brain. DIPG-Diffuse intrinsic pontine glioma.

What? No way. Not her, not us. No way.

A special surgeon was called in, he urged us to allow her to be prepped for surgery, immediately. The tumor was pressing on her spinal fluid and could leave her paralyzed if they didn't at least try to ease some pressure. We agreed. They quickly prepped her for surgery. I remember her asking me, "Yami, am I going to die?"- "Of course NOT, you'll be back to being a pain in my butt in no time". We both giggled. As they were taking her away to surgery, she said "byeee", looking back on the stretcher. "Not bye, see you later," said my older sister.

We waited for over 18 hours. You could almost see the despair in the air. We saw the surgeon approaching and he told us the surgery was a success, and as soon as she was stable, we could see her again. We all cried tears of happiness. A few hours went by, and suddenly, I heard the doctors running towards her recovery room. I heard the machines making loud noises, nurses running to her side. Oh no, the despair was back. They rushed her back to emergency surgery.

Hours later, many "deals with god" later, and the surgeon returned. The tears in his eyes were not a good sign.

Her brain had hemorrhaged, she was now declared brain dead. The world seemed different all of a sudden. Darker, grayer, confusing, meaningless. My mother had to be sedated, my father fell to his knees and begged God to take it all, his money, his businesses, his life, anything, just not his baby girl. I sat there, numb. After four days of no sleep, I looked over as my baby sister laid next to us on life support, in just a moment, life had taken a dark turn.

It took me many, many years to accept this new "normal". It took years of meaningless relationships, partying, depression and self-deprecating behavior. Five years later, the years brought me to one man, Gavin. We partied, we did drugs, we drank, we took spontaneous road trips whenever it was meant to be. We spent every day and night together. Life was starting to feel ok.

One morning, I woke up feeling just "not right". Something felt off, I couldn't shake it. Days went by, I felt out of it. Two pregnancy tests later, I was EXPECTING. That feeling of despair was back again. I didn't think I could have children, so it came as a shock to me. I told Gavin, and he was thrilled. A few nights later, I was crying in bed, he lay with me and asked me what was wrong. "I don't really believe in abortions, but if you're not ready for this, please tell me, because I am not sure if I have what it takes to be a single mom." "I will always take care of you and our baby" he assured me. The despair faded into the darkness.

I was going to be a mom, I had to learn a new way of life and unlearn my current one. As the months went by, Gavin stayed with me, most nights were great, but some nights we would get into terrible arguments about the smallest things. I would cry hysterically, those hormones and all, and he would get fed up with me and leave. One of those arguments changed everything forever. "Dramatic bitch"-he pushed me. I was about 5 months along the first time it escalated from emotional to physical abuse. It was just a one-time thing, right? We were going to be a family, I just had to learn to control the raging pregnancy hormones.

We were a family, and families stick together. As I progressed in my pregnancy, the great nights became fewer and the terrible nights became more frequent. I would check his phone after he would stay out all night and find messages to quite a few women. I would cry, he would get frustrated, push me or slap me across my mouth to "shut me up" quite often. I cried myself to sleep, almost every night.

And then, Sylar was born in August. We were so exhausted for the first 3-months that we had no time to argue. I knew everything would be just fine after those pregnancy hormones were done. We rented a new apartment, got all new furniture, and we were adulting. Gavin hadn't worked since we met. Once I found out I was pregnant, I had given him a few thousand dollars to buy sneakers, phones, anything we could sell on eBay and other sites. We made enough money for the bills, so I stayed home with Sylar and he would be out and about trying to score items to sell.

Ah, good old post-partum hormones. My body had changed, I felt innate, I felt unworthy. Gavin started staying out later and later until at one point he would only come home in the middle of the night. His phone, why did I always have to check his phone? Messages to multiple women. It was my fault, my body had changed so much, I was so tired all of the time, why would he want to be around me? I begged him to spend time with us, sending him cute pictures of the baby throughout the day, hoping he would want to come home. This went on for months, it never worked.

He came home one night, and I went crazy. Screaming at him how he was a bad boyfriend and a bad father, how I needed him, and he was nowhere to be found. He didn't take too kindly to my words. Usually, when we argued, he would slap his hand over my mouth and tell me to shut up, "we have neighbors", and keep it there until I cried and nodded to keep quiet. But this time he pushed me to the floor, yelling how I was a dog and dogs belong on the floor. I tried to get up, crying, he pushed me back down. Towering over me, he kept pushing me back down to the floor, I tasted blood. My lip was busted. "Look what you did," I cried. He disappeared for a moment and came back laughing, "You're such a LIAR, you want to talk shit, here" He tried to stuff a dirty diaper in my mouth and laughed, hysterically. "You bit your own lip so you could say I did it, do you think I'm dumb?". He dragged me by my hair across the apartment as I screamed in pain and then he let go. "I'm leaving", he yelled as he put his shoes on.

I lay on the floor, numb. A couple of hours went by, and I heard Sylar crying. I snapped back to reality and laid with him, and we fell asleep. Gavin didn't come back for a few days. It was better that way. When he finally came home, all was good again. He was being sweet, brought home food, rubbed my feet, and we fell asleep. Confusion was the best way to describe it. "This can't be happening to me. BUT we're a family, my son needs us together. I just have to lose weight and get back to my old fun self, everything will be great again. Every night could be like tonight if I was just my old self again," I thought.

Another night, another argument. He pushed me into the wall so hard I hit my head and fell down, he left me right there. The next afternoon, he called to tell me he was coming home. I told him not to dare come home, I had changed the locks. He laughed and said he's on the way. I called the police, and I assume the police cars must have scared him off because he disappeared for a few days with no word. Then the texts started rolling in, "You should kill yourself, Sylar would be better off without you", he texted. He was threatening to come back regardless, he would find a way in the apartment, he said. I packed up and went to my parents' house for a few days and when I returned, he was there. He was packing his things and a few of mine too. He took about $2,000 of my cash and I cried that that was all I had for Sylar and me. "Consider it a going away fee" he smirked and left. He had packed everything we had for sale, phones, sneakers, everything.

At that moment, I decided to move back to my parents, in shame. I felt like a failure, I was suicidal, the pain in my heart was too much to bear. I loved him and missed him so much that I felt that I couldn't breathe for weeks. He blamed me and accused me of being a traitor, I left, I broke up our family, it was all my fault because I was crazy. He told me multiple times how better off Sylar would be if I killed myself. And then something even worse happened, he blocked me on everything and changed his phone number. I couldn't reach him for roughly about three months. I wasn't sure what was worse, the overtly emotionally abusive conversations every day or the complete and utter disappearance.

"I will always take care of you and our baby"- those words he said to me, haunted me every night. How could I have been so blind? How could he have pretended all of that time to be such an amazing person? How did I allow my neediness, my self-consciousness, my self-worth to accept this? Months went by of the same, crying myself to sleep while I held my son, waking up with a hole in my heart, random texts far and in between of him telling me I was worthless, and he didn't care if I died.

During this time, I had isolated myself away from my friends and family, so I could lessen the feeling of failure. I reached out to my best friend and we cried together for hours. We came up with a plan. My son was getting older, so we made plans every day, enough to keep me busy enough to not have to think about the last few months. I started living one day at a time, sometimes just one hour at a time. That was the trick, one hour/one day at a time. As my son got older, he enjoyed different things, I would take him to the zoo, children's museums, our local toddler park, out for walks around my beautiful town's Main Street, and everything we could do to keep busy.

Little by little the hole in my chest was becoming full, I still loved him so much it physically hurt but I was starting to be able to live again. For the first time, I started to picture my future with just my son and me, and it was a happy one. Gavin did try to reach out sometimes in between those months, most times I wouldn't answer because I couldn't bear it or I would text him long paragraphs of how badly I was hurting, to which I always got a reply of "I don't care enough to read that ". After some healing, I chose to just put up with him so he could have a relationship with our son.

Months later, I was dropping off Sylar to him for the night. He was over an hour late to meet us, so he told me to use the spare key to wait inside. He hadn't seen him in a few weeks because he was "too busy". I was livid that he was an hour late to meet me, while Sylar and I just waited, I was getting angrier and angrier, I decided I was leaving, and just then, he walked in. He was high, and I said I wasn't leaving Sylar with him like that. He got angry and dragged me outside and threw me down the 5 cement steps. He locked the door, so I called 911. When he heard me on the phone, he stormed outside and took my phone and threw it down as hard as he could to smash my phone. The screen was smashed, but I could still hear the operator asking for the address, I yelled his address to her, he ran inside and locked himself in. The police arrived and after some ordeal, they retrieved Sylar from the house.

I remember my son's eyes that night, wide-eyed, staring at us, back and forth as we yelled at each other and as he dragged me away. He stuck his hand out for me as tears came down his cheeks. That was the moment. THE moment. The moment I decided I rather my son have a broken family than have to live through that, ever again. That moment I realized that I didn't deserve any of it. It wasn't my weight, my body change, my hormones, my fault at all. I didn't deserve it. I finally realized the love I had for him was toxic, I still missed my friend, the one before this all happened, but I could see now that person was gone. Periodically, he would come back into the picture trying to be a family again, I would let him spend time with our son but every time he couldn't get anything out of me, he would disappear again. New women, a new group of friends, new people to take advantage of, I was alright with that, as long as it wasn't me.

Sylar and me, just us. Sylar was about 2.5 years old and he hadn't given me a dollar. Even when I begged him months after he left me with nothing, he would laugh. I couldn't live this life. I had to be certain I would provide him with a bright future. I picked up some online classes to finally finish my degree and picked up part-time jobs to get by. I graduated and landed a great HR position with a women-owned small company. She was a major inspiration to me. Her story, her life, and her attitude proved to me that we can do it all.

Life had meaning again; I was financially stable(ish) and my son was happy. But I wanted more. Over the years after my sister had passed away, I had gone into a rabbit hole of what can affect cancer and cancerous cells, and of course, the leading factors were processed foods, chemicals in food, etc. I had forced my family to eat all organic, and make everything in-house, sazon, seasonings, everything we could make ourselves we did. And now, with more stability in my life, I could focus on what I was passionate about again.

One night while sitting on a Caribbean beach, I had this warm feeling come over me. I should start a healthy food café, with a Hispanic twist. The idea made me light up inside. I came back home from vacation on a mission. The Green Bowl- an earth-friendly, clean ingredient, café with all biodegradable containers, and authentic flavor. We range from acai bowls to salads, smoothies, rice bowls, arepas, plantain sandwiches, gluten-free empanadas and breakfast sandwiches. We have just opened our second location and the local community has fully supported us. We couldn't be more grateful.

So, you see, out of the darkest moments, comes a strength, motivation and inspiration, something like you never thought you would feel but here we are now. We don't need apologies to heal or even admittance, we know our journey, and we are what matters. My son is now 7 years old. His father is still disrespectful, helps financially very rarely and sporadically but I maintain my cool (most of the time) for Sylar's sake. But deep down, I know his abuse was a major factor in how I became as strong as I am today. It showed me that I deserved more, how I was on a self-destructive path when I met him and the pain he inflicted on me, made me choose another path in life. My son was my saving grace, I will never regret my past because it brought to me an amazing little boy who inspires me every day.

I've also launched an online store of educational toys- SyBspace.com and I am currently working on a spirituality shop with my best friend. At some point, I am also looking to bring The Green Bowl to a national level, but for now, I am plenty busy with just the two locations and the third in the works, but this is just the beginning for me. My advice to you is to take strength in your story, your pain, your tears. If you could overcome the trauma of someone who is supposed to love and protect you, betraying you in the worst way imaginable, then you can overcome anything life throws your way. You ARE strong. You ARE worthy. You ARE the light.

YAMALIT HOLGUIN

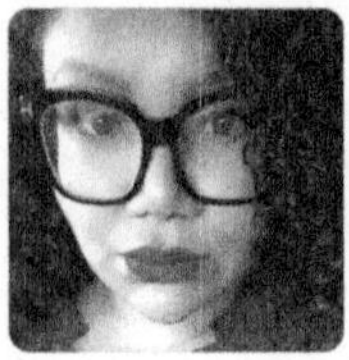

Yamalit Holguin uses her past as fuel to guide and protect her current and future paths.

After family tragedy inspired her to explore healthy eating, Yami knows our nutrition can help us fight illnesses and so switched eating habits Yami established The Green Bowl group, an eco-friendly, organic café in New York.

Yami is also the founder of SyB's Space, created to help shape our children's creativity at heart and in mind. Yami believes our children deserve better than being lost in technology day in and day out. Their minds deserve to be lit up with new ideas, amazing toys, and crafts and she is creating this online to allow international access.

It is Yami's hope that at least one person can take even a hint of inspiration from her contribution and it will be worth the pain of retelling her story.

You can connect with Yami here:
Instagram: www.instagram.com/badmamayama/
Websites: https://www.thegreenbowlny.com/
www.sybspace.com/

5

KALI JAY WALTERS

THE BRUISES FADE, BUT THE MEMORY REMAINS...

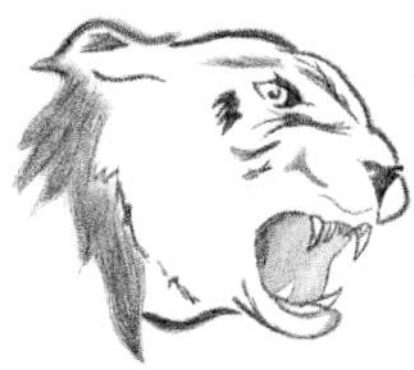

It's hard to forget the nights awake, the voices raised and the tears across your mothers' eyes. But it sort of shaped the way I viewed the world.

I am one of those children that was raised in a home of Domestic Violence, who also swore to be different but repeated the cycle until it couldn't be done anymore. This is my journey through it all in hopes that someone who needs it reads this and can escape.

Either you could be the mother, fearful that by leaving she'll mess up her kids' life, or the daughter watching on who swears she won't do the same, but is already in the pattern...

This is for you, the pain may feel real as you read it all, yet that's the thing that will give you strength to move, shift and find safety again.

Now as I look back there are so many memories that come flashing forward to me, the pieces of the puzzles that made up what I viewed life to be as a child...

- BEING THE WITNESS -

The problem with it all was that it never started off like it finished, there was a time when my father, who was the instigator of the pain, was loving and kind. He did all he could to protect and love his family. He exclaimed proudly if anyone touched his daughter he'd be the first in line.

But then it happened, not all the time at first. It started with more words than painful swings of the arms, or cracking bones and broken walls.

The yelling increased though, I can feel the fear in my body as I remember the day, the one that's started all the rest. It wasn't meant to be that way, instead, it wasn't even Dad that created this mess. It was Mum and Nana this time, arguing and fighting, yelling and screaming. It turned to much more when Dad got home though.

The sickening thud of my mothers' head hitting my father's knee, and I saw her collapse. I tried to stand in the way to save them all. But I was too small. The shame that I bore was that I somehow caused it all.

If I was bigger, if I was braver, maybe it could have ended before the crack on the skull for my mother. Her collapsing was the start of our family collapsing in a way. In a downward spiral of pain, suffering and a constant state of fear.

It's so much weight to bear as a little girl, four then, to see that pan out and make it all mean so much. But I tried to forget it and not let that be the end of the image I had of my father. How brave he was, how strong he was, my champion in the world.

I couldn't let that one time mar my image of him. Plus, Mum forgave him, so it couldn't have been that bad right?

Right from that moment, she showed me that if a man apologized and showed he was truly sorry then the pain didn't matter. She showed me that a man could hit a woman if the woman does something wrong. Grooming my image of how relationships were supposed to be and what the roles truly looked like.

I feel I need to fast forward this awhile because after that first it was hidden again, or at least the fist, the moments of rage and the physical abuse was. I still woke up to hearing them arguing, or at least hearing my father scream abuse. And I would sneak out of my room and see Mum cowered in the corner, Dad over her screaming and yelling. I'd whimper and he'd turn, he'd calm down and mildly tell me "Go back to bed..."

The next time it hit so hard and he hit harder, was a few years later. No, it didn't just stop and then come back, it was more that he was busy working, being a true horseman and someone I was proud of by day, but someone I hid from at night.

I'm sorry Mum for not protecting you in those times, maybe that's why it became harder for you to protect me when it turned around.

By the time I was seven we'd moved twice more, and now we lived in the middle of nowhere out Coonamble way, in New South Wales, Australia.

I was used to hearing the shouting by now, it almost felt normal, like it needed to happen for me to go to sleep. I had conditioned myself to not only hear him shouting at her, but in his rage he'd come into my room and scream abuse at me too while I winced and pretended to sleep. That was, until my Nana came and stopped him every time. She was a strong woman at that time. Unfortunately, it wore her down as the years went on.

Back to Coonamble though, this was where it really got worse and the true Jekyll & Hyde that is my father, came out. I now had no escape living so far out of town, I was now distance educated and surrounded by the pain of it all permanently.

I heard every hit, saw every tear, felt every word of her being torn down. Inside my childhood had been stripped of me already from these moments and from sexual abuse I experienced the year before. Yet now I was the child surrounded by it all and all I wanted to do was fix it. I'd never seen it this bad before, I thought it was all my fault that if I wasn't at home they wouldn't be feeling this bad.

It's funny being that child, how much you absorb when the mother thinks that if she stays it's best for the child, so she stays not realising the pain the child really feels inside.

Now, though it escalated, I watched one night them both out the back. My mother begged for her life while I crept and looked through the backdoor. There my father was choking her. I really thought he had killed her this time. He laid her down, and suddenly, I saw him weeping and begging "don't be dead, oh don't be dead..." He started compressions and mouth to mouth, then just hugged her and carried her towards the house.

I ran back to my room, too scared to face off with what could have been the end that night. My little mind was still so confused and wondering why, why did he keep doing this, what was so wrong, wasn't he sorry, wasn't he my hero...? It must have been me, I was the problem. He saw me when he looked at her, and in that he wanted me gone.

Maybe if I had cried and screamed, instead of staying silent but I was too afraid...

The next morning though, she was there with what I see in my memories now, the broken smile. The smile of a woman who lost herself and at that time she wouldn't have been found. No one said a word about that night, but it laid in my heart for years after that.

As the years went on every day became something new, and each time there was a new excuse, a new reason why she was to blame... The next time I saw him walk away at almost killing point because I made a noise, this time though it was day time as the abuse had moved from hidden, to plain sight.

He walked out though, and she begged for him to come back, he kept on walking... I thought I was helping and wrote two notes, one for him, and one for her...

"Daddy, I'm sorry I don't know what I did to make you so angry at Mummy, but please come back she loves you very much and needs you around".

"Mummy, I'm sorry I pushed Daddy away, I'll try better next time, I will get him back for you".

He yelled at me, and she just cried. He told me to "fuck off", confirming it was my fault. And she just cried...

But he stayed. In hindsight, I wish he would have gone now, maybe then life wouldn't have taken the painful route it did. But then again, on my side, I wouldn't have had the strength I have to keep on going and keep moving forward with life... Who knows?

I witnessed again as a child, what a relationship looked like and believed that it was something normal. Even though Mum would hide the scars from others and it was in hushed whispers... I thought that it was one of those things that happened to everyone because it's all I knew.

After this, though I was no longer just the child witnessing it, I became a part of it. I put myself in the middle of it and got hurt time and time again, for her, by him. By her, for herself. She had the "hurt people... hurt people" side coming through.

It taught me so much, but most of all, what was meant to be unconditional love. What a painful thing to learn in this way...

I was eleven when that rifle was pulled, he told her he would shoot me if she didn't stop screaming. I pleaded with my eyes, "please

Mum, please be quiet", fearing I would die that night. She dulled and went to a whisper. I was saved that time...

That rifle was pulled again and again, the scare tactic, because none of us knew exactly what he would do. He was crazy and neurotic. He loved us, he hated us, he wished we were dead, we were his world.

When I was fourteen I stood up with my mother, as he fired at her, missing by centimetres, above her head. The only reason we were spared was because of being so scared we dropped a little to the ground.

He cursed her and threw me aside on a lounge. I sat there quivering not knowing what to do. I started getting angry though. By now, I was using drugs, smoking and drinking too.

Anything to numb the pain as my life became not just a witness to, but also an experiencer of the pain.

He started to kick us out, and I saw my mother beg to stay, so I dropped to my knees and begged with her too... Please let us stay at least till morning.

It's a funny thing what fear will make you do... I begged, I pleaded, and I made the deal for her. She had lost her words; it was me creating the moments. I felt twisted inside, I felt the knots boil up. I didn't want to be here anymore, but I couldn't go against her, I couldn't leave her.

> "Children hear everything you say, and they mimic everything you do... So, choose your words and actions carefully..."
>
> — SUSHMA JAKHAR

- BECOMING THE ONE TO EXPERIENCE IT TOO -

At sixteen I had my first true boyfriend, a long-distance one at that. I latched on to the first person who gave me the attention, the first person who was a male that showed that they loved me. Turns out I chose wrong. He never would hit me, which I just said made it okay.

The mental abuse that he put me through, the twisted-up stories and the suicidal pieces, I couldn't break up with him or he would die. He would make sure I messaged at specific times, and if I didn't wow, would I be shown how useless I truly was. How much of a problem I was...

By seventeen I had been kicked out of home, scared for my life I went into a women's refuge. And there I felt empowered enough to break up with my first boyfriend.

When my father almost killed me, it was time to leave my much-loved town. I moved across to be with someone I'd known for a while and thought that he was decent. He swore never to hit a woman and sure, he protected me. I was so protected that he made sure I was under his watch every step of the way. Controlling and manipulating my scared little heart.

We broke up not long after that, and it led to my next step in the cycle. One of the worst people I had been with was the one that started to hurt me, he would throw things and hit me. I said to myself it's not so bad, at least he never tried to kill me.

I think that because I was using heavier than ever before, I now disconnected myself from the pain. I told myself I deserved it, repeated the words no man would ever want me. Reconfirmed by the pain. Reconfirmed by the breakups...

I thought I then met my Knight in shining armour... but instead, he was just another abuser in tin foil.

He was blonde with blue eyes, and he had a nice smile. It seemed so wonderful he cared, he loved me, he did all things right. But it didn't last long till the voices were raised and I started to feel scared all over again.

My light had died inside. I had gotten to the point of hearing all the words repeated from him, that Dad had said to Mum, had said to me. I was worthless, useless and didn't deserve it.

I flinched as he spoke. He threw things and that would almost hit me, but then he laid hands on me and claims it never happened. He said I must not remember correctly, or I was too high, but the bruising explained it. The pain and the memories never truly faded.

I wanted to break the cycle, but it never happened. I felt weak and useless. Everything I had been told I was.

I was using to numb the pain, he was always telling me that I was remembering wrong. While keeping me on a short leash.

- ENOUGH IS ENOUGH, IT'S TIME TO RISE ABOVE -

We both ended up going to rehab and I started to see things without the numbing of drugs. I started to remember the times as I shrank from his fists, or silently laid there and took it as he sexually abused me, too scared to say anything in case I got hurt from it.

The moments I saw as weaknesses turned to moments of courage as I witnessed myself through new eyes.

The moments I questioned whether I made it all up turned to moments of knowing as I felt my own pain...

I found out I was pregnant, and even though I wanted to run at first I stayed. Until I couldn't anymore, until I replayed enough to decide that enough is enough.

I couldn't let her go through it all the same as I had. I knew no one would touch me again, I wasn't going to allow it.

After we had broken up there was one phone call that completely changed me... He told me in a fit of anger "I'm going to stomp your head in, I want you DEAD!"

I was scared again, but all that had led me to this point reminded me that I could and would survive. I was strategic in some of my ways, keeping in safe spaces and creating exchanges with him that couldn't be any other way but documented.

There comes a time when the line in the sand is drawn and we never go back... THIS WAS MINE!

I rekindled a romance with an old school sweetheart, but I kept my heart kind of barricaded, loving him yet not fully trusting.

I looked out for the red flags this time. This time I was not going to allow the cycle to keep repeating.

I started to speak even when my voice shook. I started to put up boundaries even if they came from fear, they were my protected boundaries and were clear.

I found my self-worth and started to see myself differently as I listened to words of kindness, from myself not from a man.

It's been ten years this year since I last heard an abuser's voice threaten to hurt me. As each year goes by I remember I am not just a survivor. I am the heroine in my journey. I broke the pattern because I saw that I needed to be more, for myself, for my child.

To the child I was, it was never your fault. To the woman I grew to be, good work for living. To the woman I am now, I am so proud of you...

Look where you got to, now inspiring women who were shown dysfunction, and their inner child wounded. Look at what you're building, even though you thought you were broken.

I know that the wounds, the bruises and the physical pain is gone, but the memories are still there... Funny though, as I wrote these words it let go of some of that pain, some of that strain.

To my sistah reading this, don't stay for the children, they want to see you shine too. Don't stay for the child because you think they deserve to be in a whole family. Go for yourself, so they can see your strength shine. Go for yourself, it's not worth your life.

To my sistah reading this, don't beat yourself up, the patterns were shown to you deep through your line. Don't try to discourage your strength, it's truly shining. Stand strong in your power, show tears if you've got them.

But rise up my dear sistah and go for yourself. I know the fear of looking behind you hoping they won't find you. But rise up dear sistah and keep on shining.

KALI JAY WALTERS

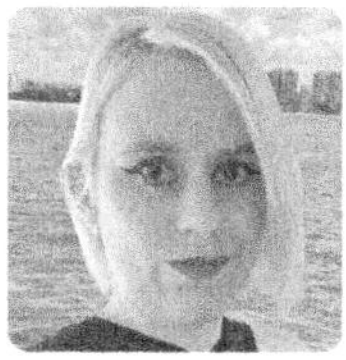

After living a life of abuse and trauma in her childhood, Kali J fell into a state of addiction and repeating the cycles of abuse she saw before her. Kali J found her way out of it all by saying enough was enough and creating differently in her life.

Now Kali Jay has five children, a loving husband, and is living a passion-filled life by healing and learning how to shift her world.

Kali Jay coaches women to take their power back, clearing the anger and fear that has restricted them in life, showing them to break free and claim their permission to shine again. Kali Jay hosts a free group, The Mummas Permission Movement for mums to come together and rise with celebration, ceremony and complete safety.

Kali J would love to have you connect with her at:
Website: www.kalijwalters.com
Facebook: www.facebook.com/KaliJWalters55
The Mummas Permission Movement:
www.facebook.com/groups/mpmovement/

6

SHEILA KADEER

SATURDAY IS NOT A GOOD DAY TO DIE

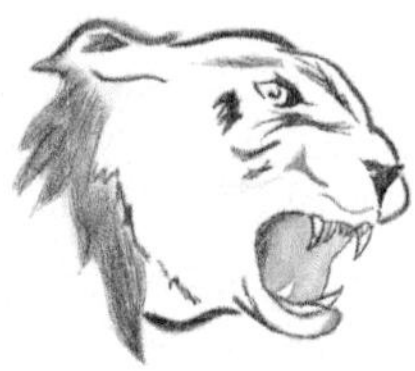

The baseball bat skimmed past my legs as he swung it at me. The anger and rage contorting the features of his face. Pure venom and hate directed at me. How dare I challenge him. How dare I question him about his affair. Four years of abuse and THIS is how it was going to end? By beating me to death with a baseball bat on a sunny Saturday afternoon? Leaving my three-year-old daughter to live a life with HIM. No fucking way.

I didn't know he had brought the baseball bat into the house. I didn't know he even had one, let alone was keeping it in the boot of his car. But he did. For four years I was verbally, physically and mentally abused. No one knew. Why would they? I never told anyone. I kept it all to myself. I had a good job and I earned good money. As the police would later say, we were Mr and Mrs Respectable. The thing is you don't know what goes on behind closed doors. To the outside world, we were the perfect couple. Nice house, adorable child, all the trappings of success. But the reality was so different.

Over the four years I stayed with him, I had a knife put to my throat and stomach while I was pregnant. I had been kicked and beaten on the floor while I tried to protect my face in front of my baby, punched in the face, had car keys hidden so I couldn't leave, phone line pulled out, and even contact lenses and glasses taken away so I couldn't even see, my food spat in. Violence and abuse was an everyday occurrence.

Each day I came home in fear, not knowing what mood he may be in. So why didn't I leave? The thing is I could not leave because he controlled access to my daughter. His mother looked after her while we both worked. He picked her up every day. His mother knew what was going on, I am sure of it but I would not have been allowed to leave the relationship with my daughter. I knew this, so I had to stay to protect her.

On the day of the baseball bat incident, I told him I knew he was having an affair and I wanted us to split up. This was not how things were going to play out by his rules. He wanted me out of the way so he could move his latest conquest in and keep my daughter. He knew this day would come and he prepared well for it. He opened the cupboard and grabbed the bat that he had recently brought in from his car. As I saw it, I tried to shut the door on his hand, it gave me a few seconds to start running towards the back of the house. Everything was in slow motion. The back door was locked and the keys were gone. Oh, how he had planned this day.

My daughter ran and hid under a table, her safe place when the violence was happening. Watching silently and taking it all in. Standing at the back door in desperation a soft voice spoke to me and said "the key is above the ledge". I really believe this was an angel. She knew it was not my time to die, I had work to do. I fumbled for the key and opened the door with him in hot pursuit. Now outside in the garden, I could scream as loud as I could for help. This stopped him in his tracks. He ran back into the house, grabbed my daughter, jumped in his car and left.

As soon as I saw the car go, I ran back inside and called my parents. This was the first time I had told anyone what was going on. They called the police. While they were talking to me, he came back. He was arrested for attempted murder and bundled into the back of a police car and taken away. It's finally over, I thought to myself.

He was let out the next day and no charges were ever brought. He was allowed to come back to the house. I had no protection. Thus began my long journey with the civil courts. Before the baseball bat incident, I had already seen a solicitor for advice on leaving, splitting the house and shared custody of our child. I knew he was having an affair and I was preparing for what I hoped would be an amicable split based on the fact there was someone else involved. A letter came to the house, addressed to me, from my solicitor which he opened and took. It detailed how much would be a fair amount to offer him to leave the house and the fairest way forward for custody and contact with our daughter. This is where things began to spiral as he was losing control, he could no longer have it all his own way.

I started court proceedings beginning with a non-molestation injunction. I went to live with my mum and took my daughter there. He was offered visitation at a contact centre. He started to harass me at work, I had phone calls and many threats to my life. He demanded I pay him £20,000 and if I did, he would walk away from everything and have nothing to do with our daughter. My father and I tried to raise the money. We offered him the money and he then told me the price had gone up to £40,000. I told him no, I could not get £40,000.

He then started proceedings against me for full custody. This would become almost a year of hell. Every time my daughter came back from visits with him, she was upset, angry and we'd have major behavioural issues.

The lies started. He started to say I was a bad mother, that I was the violent one, that I was abusing my daughter. I started to keep a log of everything. Every abusive phone call I got, everything my daughter said after visits. As with all cases involving children, the appropriate organisations were placed to help the court case and investigate. He was such a good liar, manipulative and believable, he could make them doubt me and think that I'm crazy.

We got a court date for custody. He lied all the way through. I was painted as a vindictive woman who was jealous about him having an affair and was making up the violence for revenge. His barrister tore me to pieces. The judgement was made. He should live in the house, as he worked from home, and he would have interim custody. I was given visits on Mondays and Wednesdays for two hours in the evening. WHAT THE ACTUAL FUCK!? What kind of legal system takes a child away from the mother and gives her to a violent man? With tears in my eyes I asked my solicitor "please do something". She looked as shocked as me but was powerless to do anything. The decision was made.

I was distraught and cried all night. My daughter was screaming "NO MUMMY I DON'T WANT TO GO" as my father tried to get her into the car to take her to him. THIS IS NOT RIGHT. My life had fallen apart. I had a choice, give up and let him win or FUCKING ROAR.

I chose to ROAR. I was given a date to go to MY house that I still paid the mortgage on and bills, to pick my belongings. His mother and father were there while my parents and I tried to gather as much of my personal belongings as possible. His mother smirked at me. I will never forget that "this is not a fucking game lady, this is my child's life". I so desperately wanted to tell her what we were doing. Being a woman who ROARS, I was going to high court to get this decision by a delusional judge overturned. I was told not to give the game away, but it was so bloody hard.

While he was living in the house, he moved in his seventeen-year-old girlfriend. He had been told she must not have anything to do with our child. We know this because my daughter told me. He played a good game. But I learnt to play it better, so I hired a private investigator. We got photographic evidence of his girlfriend hiding in the footwell of the car and getting out and running in the house. Yes, she actually crouched down in the footwell so she could not be seen in the car driving up the road. Unbelievable.

My daughter started to divulge witnessing sexual acts and being left on her own in the house while he took his girlfriend to work. I cannot believe our justice system has allowed this to happen. But I was unable to do a damn thing.

I was supposed to be keeping all the evidence to myself until the final court case. I was talking to the social worker about my concerns and I knew she didn't believe me. He had manipulated her so much. So I blurted out, "I have photos of the girlfriend at the house'. She was shocked. She wanted to see them right away. She made an emergency appointment to see my solicitor and she was shown the photos. Now she saw the truth, she couldn't believe she had been hoodwinked and manipulated.

After a wait to get a date, we finally went to High Court. We won. It was overturned. They said this should never have happened and the original judge was absolutely wrong. He was taken off the case and a more senior judge appointed. I was overjoyed but I knew it was not the end as interim custody reverted to me and I was told I can live in the house and he must leave. He was granted contact though. He didn't leave quietly, in revenge he took a lot of my personal belongings and he even took the TV so my daughter couldn't watch it.

The next time I saw him was in court. It was a preliminary hearing. He was trying to get something changed or back in the house or the old judge back. I don't remember the exact details as it was over 20 years ago now. His barrister got up to speak. I now had a barrister too. After an angel spoke to me and helped me live through the baseball incident I became curious and wondered if they could help me in court. I asked Archangel Michael, Gabriel, Raphael and Uriel to stand in each corner of the courtroom. I asked Archangel Gabriel, the Archangel of Communication, to stand next to his barrister. I asked that only truth could come out of his mouth. What happened next astounded me. I still giggle about this now. Well, he could not speak. He was talking absolute gibberish. It was like a scene from the Jim Carey film Bruce Almighty. Everyone just looked at him like he was a blithering idiot. We never saw him again, my ex stopped paying his legal bills and he represented himself from then on in.

LET BATTLE COMMENCE.

He continued to lie throughout the case, bringing me back to court and incurring fees for me. He had no fees anymore as he represented himself. He was trying to manipulate everyone. He was very convincing and so I continued to gather my evidence.

My solicitors approached the neighbours for statements. They were reluctant to get involved but we did get some statements. One of my neighbours had very interesting information that I had no idea was happening. After I'd been ordered to leave by the first judge, he was outside in the garden with my daughter one day. The neighbour heard him saying "Mummy hits you doesn't she, say it, say Mummy hits you." He was saying this over and over again to brainwash her to believe this was true and to say it to the social worker. I feel so guilty that she had been treated this way.

The last bit of evidence we needed was from an ex-girlfriend. He was with her before me and had a daughter with her. He told me that he was not allowed to see the daughter because the mother and family were being vindictive. I reached out to her when the order was made for my daughter to live with him. I was desperate for help. She did not want to get involved but eventually agreed to talk to me. She told me of her own battles with him, they had been to court, he eventually agreed to go away if she did not apply for any maintenance. She spoke about how he pushed her down the stairs when she was pregnant. She spoke about the violence, the rages and her fear. All too familiar.

My solicitor got a statement from her. She said she did not want to go to court as she did not want to see him, so we had to witness summons her, which meant she had to attend and give evidence, or she would be in contempt of court. I had to prove beyond a shadow of a doubt that I was telling the truth and he was violent and everything that came out of his mouth was a lie.

THE FINAL COURT CASE.

I sat in the court witness waiting room with my family until I was called into court. His family was there. We sat through abuse and nasty comments from them. I just sat quietly and wrote down everything they said. They actually said we must be bribing the judge. I gave my written notes to my barrister as we went in. She read them out to the judge. I think he got a picture of what we were dealing with.

I took the stand to give evidence. He started to question me, thinking he was some hot shot lawyer, you could clearly see the anger in his face. He called me a liar, that I was making things up. How come I could remember the details of the abuse but not other non-relevant details, he shouted. I looked him directly in the eye and said, "the violent episodes are etched in my memory and I will never forget them". I turned to the judge with tears in my eyes and said "I am sorry I can't do this anymore, the way he is looking at me, the evil in his face, what you are witnessing right there, that is what my life was like every day."

The judge ordered a cup of tea brought to me in the dock and that I have a break before continuing. Witness statements were read out and you could see the judge looking at me, then at him. The ex-girlfriend took the stand. She told a story, not dissimilar to mine. He cross-examined her and told her she was lying. She looked at him and said "this case has nothing to do with me, I have no reason to lie, I have nothing to gain. This is the truth and this is what you did to me." Her evidence was compelling, a final nail in the coffin.

On the last day of court I presented to my barrister a recording I had made on a dictaphone of the day the first judge had ordered us to live together but in separate rooms, this was before this judge had ordered me out of my home. He thought it would be a good idea for us to just have separate rooms first. I am not sure what planet this judge was living on, but it certainly wasn't Earth. "My family is in the house and we are putting a lock on my bedroom door. He is making verbal threats to have me killed and that I will not make it through any court case". My daughter can be heard in the background pleading with him "Daddy no, stop it, please."

It is played in court, the judge wanted to listen to it a few times as he couldn't quite believe what he was hearing. He tried a different angle. He tried to make out I was just after money. He then produced the letter my solicitor sent me when I first sought help on leaving him. My barrister snatched it off him and stated this is a privileged document that you took and should not have.

The case closed for the judge to make his decision. Judgement day finally arrived, and I sat in the courtroom feeling sick to my stomach. The judge started to speak. We had findings of fact that he was violent. That what I said was TRUE. "I am finally believed". He was ordered to pay my costs because he was found to be being vindictive and incurring costs for me the whole way through. He was also given a no direct contact order which meant that he should have no contact with our daughter.

I would shake for years after just at the thought of him. There are way too many memories of violence and mental abuse and I still get triggers now some 20 years later. My daughter had trauma therapy for the violence she witnessed, she has also had counselling as a young adult to help deal with her anxiety.

Because of the lack of help and support I received I decided to become a police officer. This was a way for me to take my power back, to be in authority and help other people. I joined in 2014, leaving a successful corporate career and taking a 50% pay cut to do so. I felt it so strongly though, I needed to do it.

It was really hard to get in, I failed the fitness test the first time and had to train hard to get to the level required. I even went as far as getting laser eye surgery so that I could meet the eyesight requirements. I was determined to get in. I am so grateful and proud that I became a police officer. I loved my job. I went to so many domestic abuse incidents and was able to help so many women. Giving them the help I never got. Believing them and being there for them. I became one of the first specially trained officers for the force helping women who had been raped or sexually assaulted.

Unfortunately, while I was doing that role my father died suddenly. I suffered depression and needed to take a career break to heal. I did go back some four years later but burnt out after about 18 months so left once and for all and actually became a private investigator for a while! Helping women from a different angle and gathering evidence for them, just like the investigator I used all those years ago.

WHAT DID THIS TEACH ME?

Through all of this, I never gave up. The truth will always come out. Even when the odds are stacked against you, keep believing in yourself. Yes, it may be hard but you have to keep going. When you are dealing with narcissists you have to learn to think like them and be one step ahead. I collated notes of every threatening call, everything that was said and I produced this in court. Every time I was told I was lying I could go to the scrap of paper for that event and say what was said or done.

When someone takes away your power, do what you need to do to take it back. For me it was joining the police, for you it might be moving to a new city, or taking a new job or just saying NO. I was so proud to be a police officer, I would never have achieved this if I was not pushed to my limits. One of the little things I did for myself straight after was get my hair done, he would become abusive just because I wanted to buy hair conditioner! So this little step helped me take back my power too.

You cannot change the past, but you can change your future. Just because things have been difficult in the past, it does not mean you cannot create a beautiful future. I have moved past the anger, bitterness and hurt and I fully accept what happened. It has changed my life but in a way, I did not expect. I have gone down a path that allows me to transform other people's lives and it makes me feel alive.

I will continue to ROAR for myself, my daughter and all the women I will help in the future.

SHEILA KADEER

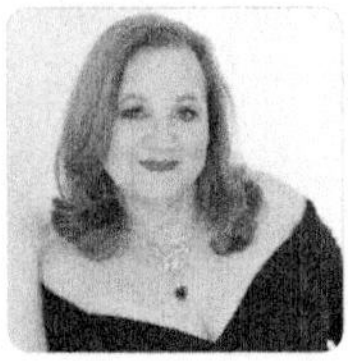

Sheila Kadeer is an Intuitive Business Coach based in the UK. For four years Sheila and her daughter were locked in a cycle of domestic abuse, culminating in a long court battle with her abuser.

After winning her court case she made it her mission to support other women going through domestic abuse. She became a police officer and later a Specially Trained Officer dealing with victims of serious sexual assault and rape.

The sudden death of her father leading to depression, called Sheila to begin her own journey to heal from the pain of her past. Sheila now works with spiritual entrepreneurs to clear the core wounds that are holding them back from elevating to their next level income and impact so that they can magnetically attract abundance and create an extraordinary life that brings them deep fulfilment and freedom.

When she is not working she can be found walking the countryside with her dog 'Musky the Husky'.

Website: www.sheilakadeer.com

Facebook: www.facebook.com/SheilaKadeerBoldBusinessWitch

Instagram: www.instagram.com/sheila.kadeer/

7

YVONNE MUNDIH

UNIQUE LIFE STORY

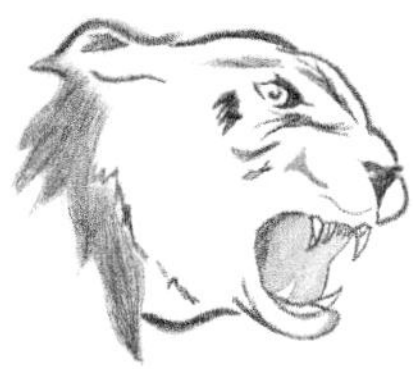

"A woman in harmony with her spirit is like a river flowing.

She goes where she will without pretence and arrives at her destination

Prepared to be herself and only herself."

— MAYA ANGELOU

It was many years ago. Yet it seems so fresh within me like a new wound just opened up. Writing this chapter has re-ignited in me the sleeping dog that lay. This chapter is the beginning of so many years and layers of pain that have over the years sought for that voice, pen and paper of expression to continue to heal and to heal others.

A GRANDMOTHER'S MANTLE

No matter life's circumstances, life is a continuous fight to conquer and to build on New territories for the one who dares to say, I can and I will.

Use your inner gifts to build monuments in places where

STARS are born out of scars.

I always knew there was something different about me, my mother and my siblings. I was trapped in a biological father's home.

I worked hard to earn his affection and approval. This took me into various abusive situations up until adulthood, still trying to earn his affection and approval until he passed in 2018. You could call it a severe case of domestic abuse.

My ordeal started with a mother who was given away in marriage at 16. After two years of marriage, a rapid wave and storm of events came against her.

Shortly after she gave birth to beautiful twin girls, her husband was killed, her property seized, and she was raped in the filthiest way while still breastfeeding her twin babies. Pregnant with me, she was forced to live with her 59-year-old abuser in his compound, amongst his wives and children with some around her age.

She was only 18 at the time. She ended up with nine children of her own. Six are no more due to abuse and depression, and two brothers are addicted to alcohol to try to dull their pain.

I was born and raised in a patriarchal system. A system in which men hold primary power and predominate in roles of political leadership, moral authority, social privilege and control of property. The woman's role is relegated to the kitchen, childbearing, domestic chores and satisfying the man.

The female child stands to suffer as she is deprived of education, forced into marriage at a young age, and is made to accept male dominance in all areas without question. Domestic violence against women and children, particularly female children is predominant.

The female child is seen as property to be sold in marriage, thus violating the much-cherished tradition of Bride Price for the sake of protection.

At three, my father gave me away against the pleas and cries of my mother. Away in a distant land, my mother stealthily visited me once in eight years.

The good news is that even though I had a difficult time, I was sent to primary school, an indication of hope for mental freedom.

"The educated mind is a free mind" in the words of my mother. She always reminds me of how blind she is due to her inability to read and write.

By the time I was 15, I had lived in multiple different homes in which I suffered tremendous abuse and rejection. **I don't know why I was born, but I guess everything that happened to me, happened for me.**

I graduated from primary school at the age of 11. A few weeks later, my father demanded that I be sent to the village.

My arrival in the village was the beginning of my confidence in my grandmother's belief that a strong woman is shaped by life's circumstances. She gathers her courage and discipline from harsh things thrown at her repeatedly. And above all, a warrior child is born out of the scars it bears along the journey of life.

I was put under fear, self-doubt, and confusion.

I have learned that life is full of a mixture of adventures.

It is our ATTITUDE towards it that determines which way we go.

My unique story is about the storms I faced in life, yet with determination, I found a voice, a pen and paper, love and care for others among other things to become and thrive in spite of.

The spirit of my grandmother, through a traditional ritual blessing, is in me and will always push me on to climb higher mountains, build monuments and be all that God has created me to be. There is nothing that I cannot do.

She taught me that **"if there is no enemy within you the enemy outside can do you no harm."**

I AM 11 YEARS OLD.

Sitting in the kitchen surrounded by my brothers, grandmother and father.

My father in anger tells my grandmother he wants me to get married to a man of his choice.

Dead silence fills the kitchen.

"Do you hear me?" My father reiterated.

More dead silence and fear gripped me and the food in my mouth turned bitter.

Reflecting over the years, my grandmother humbly told my father how disappointed she was in the way my mother and her children were treated.

She told my father that my granddaughter was too young to get married.

I would like her to be educated like your older girls as well.

What followed this conversation almost left my grandmother dead if my brother had not sneaked out to summon an elderly neighbor.

In spite of all this, my grandmother was determined to give away her life to save mine.

My father never loved me.

He arranged for me to marry a 38-year-old man I didn't know nor love.

He told me "**Mundih, unless you do what I ask you, you will never amount to anything, you will sleep in the bush with animals.**"

I could not understand why my father hated me so much.

I contemplated suicide and actually prayed to God to take my mother and her children, or at least me.

When my grandmother left, at midnight my father sent me out into the dark.

I groped my way around the village to a neighbor's house.

With a lighted bush lamp, the neighbor took me across the river to my grandmother.

My father found out and threatened the entire village to never take me in.

This was my new lifestyle for months.

The bush became my home.

Hunger, fear, and dirt infested me.

Most of the time, my mother was on the run for her dear life.

On their way to the farm early in the morning, the village women would stealthily and kindly drop food on plantain leaves for me.

I wandered around during the day to find palm kernels and fruits to eat if the village women did not bring me food.

I was lonely and terrified.

At one point, I went on a hunger strike, cried all night and day, hoping to die.

I felt treated unfairly.

Then one day, an elderly neighbor asked to take me to the city to be a housekeeper.

My father told him, "take her, I don't care."

After about a year as a housekeeper, my father again ordered that I be sent to the village to get married.

I was 12 years old now.

Back in the village, though unhappy, I was glad I was back to protect my mother and my siblings.

I had this dream of building a beautiful home for my mom.

One day I asked my mom if we could run away from my father to a distant village for refuge.

Her answer was in her sobs as she raised her hands to the spirit of our ancestors in prayer.

Deeply she told me **"My daughter, the horse that does not have a tail, it is only God who sends its flies away"**. Metaphorical and loaded.

At this point, I began to search my soul and ask a series of questions.

Why my mother and her children? Why me?

I felt more rejection and started believing in the paradigms inside of me that I truly would never amount to anything.

The bitterness against my father grew.

One day, my father loaded a gun to shoot my mother.

Behold, the Spirit of my ancestors was at work. Somehow my mom had been removed from our one-bedroom house. He fired the gun in her room and left.

At this point, I began to question my existence.

I began to isolate myself.

I became too quiet.

This took a toll on my mother and my siblings who were very afraid of what my father was capable of doing.

My mom became disoriented.

With no one to protect us, I told myself that I deserve better for me, my mom, siblings, and not just to please my father.

I decided to do whatever it took to stand and to succeed in life.

I was determined to be educated to improve my life.

My mom was unable to pay my way to school.

I decided to do farming, selling vegetables, and other small businesses.

I was enrolled in secondary school the following year at 13. Exciting!

I admired the style of the educated so much.

After secondary school, I decided to go to high school. With fear, my mother enrolled me.

My suffering reminded me of my grandmother's teachings:

"There has not been any truly happy and successful person with an easy past."

"Without any pain, there will be no gain in life."

"You are a child of our ancestors and The spirit God, and no weapon fashioned against you shall prosper". Psalm 91 was and is still my shield and comfort.

I graduated from high school with flying colors.

I decided to attend university.

My mom became very sceptical.

She said: "**My daughter, I want you to be highly educated because I never went to school. But our problems might get worse because you will become the first female child of this village to attend higher education.**"

All I wanted was to better my life and that of my mom and siblings.

Behold, the spirit of my ancestors was on my side.

The loving parents of this village came together in kind and cash and decided to educate me further.

"ONE GOOD TURN DESERVES ANOTHER."

I spent most of my holidays in the village, reading, writing, doing community work, cooking for the old and the young, teaching Sunday school and writing letters for the parents of the village.

I became the village courier.

I have come to understand that if you don't fight for what you want, what you don't want will automatically kick in for you.

I graduated and became the very first female child in the village for more than ten years with a bachelor's degree. Amazing!

I was grateful!

The spirit of a warrior grandmother reigns in me.

Life is hard, but I have learned to play it with determination to win it.

"THE ONE WHO IS DETERMINED TO WIN IS THE ONE WHO MAKES BREAKTHROUGHS."

I was determined to be the first to eliminate abuse, rejection, poverty, homelessness, hunger, fear and squalor in my family. And it's happening.

My grandmother's spirit, my mother, and the Universe paved a way for me where I was denied.

One time I went to watch TV with the only TV owner in the village. He talked about freedom and success in America.

I became so obsessed with coming to America that I almost went insane.

My grandmother prayed and told me that the big bird flying in the sky will take me to America. I believed her.

I was humbled, writing from that place of freedom in the United States of America. **"Freedom denied is freedom given."**

Still, in search of love and acceptance, I got married twice within five years to men I thought I loved. Within a year into both relationships, I realized that I made bad choices. Both became exploitative, psychologically, emotionally, and physically abusive.

I ended up with two divorces. A reflection of my father, it seems.

It just seemed natural that you get attracted to the same kind of people to the way your father treated you as a child.

The paradigms in my head played over and over again.

I felt like I made the wrong choices just to please somebody else.

It felt like I was at the end of a cul de sac.

I learned that where there is a will, there is a way. And sometimes when things begin to shake in our lives, it is actually our spirit

ancestors that are doing the shaking in order to thrust us to better destinations. I was determined to conquer, reign, and build an Empire for myself.

As I struggled, there was something in me that said I will overcome and thrive like others.

Then all of a sudden, my powerful spirit, mentor, protector grandmother passed.

My two brothers also passed leaving behind little angels.

One biological and nine adopted children, including my sick mother rested on my shoulders.

I invited my mother. She was diagnosed with a stomach aneurysm and was ordered for immediate surgery or else she would die.

A big down payment awaited me as she had no insurance.

I began a ritual of gratefulness in all situations and I took pride in the fact that I am still standing. I began to believe that out of my storms came purpose and hope for others. I thought about the traditional ritual blessing of my grandmother, the lessons and my dreams buried in a plastic bag. A spiritual warrior child rose up in me and said your spirit God is with you.

I thought about how far I have come in life.

I believe that God has a Divine appointment and purpose for my life. I thought about other girls who suffered the same fate as me and are no more, especially one little girl who died of abuse at the age of 8. My mother tried adopting her and her father refused.

Haunted by the spirit of my siblings and this little girl, my Mission now is to speak and advocate for the abused, rejected, the poor, hungry, homeless, abandoned, those pushed to the backwaters of life for no fault of their own, particularly women and children. Domestic abuse is my emblem for life.

Even though I was beaten and left to die, my journals seized and burnt, I was determined to help.

I cried out to my spirit creator.

One Sunday, in tears, a flash of light went through my mind. My grandmother's voice appeared to me and said: "**Stand up and wipe your tears, it's getting better for you, be a MANTLE.**"

I started googling information seminars. I found two including The Les Brown Power Voice Academy. I attended and graduated.

My voice, pen and paper, and the determined spirit of a warrior have been the weapons I have.

The beginning of my journey of personal growth.

Then my breakthrough came. A friend invited me to join a speaker and coach training.

I took a leap of faith and joined.

I took a bigger leap of faith and invested money borrowed from my son. I am grateful for my son. Amazing son! I am now dancing in my own greatness.

My life took a different turn entirely.

I feel a kind of unexplainable spirit of excitement within me.

I am now an Internationally published author, co-author of three more books coming up soon. And I have been invited to speak at the International Women Leadership and Wellness Expo in France for 2022.

My topic is "Child Marriage." Domestic violence has to stop.

My mission now is to speak, coach, teach, write and help others, particularly women and children to do the same, and to be warriors of success in their own natural right.

Living their lives from an emotional, inner and spiritual point rather than what the world has to dictate to them.

I have learned throughout my amazing journey to not look down on myself just because of what someone wants, thinks, does, or says about me.

In the storms of relationships and life, keep humble, believe in your inner spirit to thrive and not just survive.

If you are looking for a soul transformation and to find your purpose and vision for your life, I am here to help.

If you are looking for speakers, coaches, teachers, crafting your unique story, or needing tools or a voice to uplift you from situations you cannot navigate alone, I am here to help.

If you want to open up your mind to new opportunities or be a better leader in your own life, your children, or your business, I can help.

As a child, I didn't understand. Yes as an adult, I have gotten off course several times after rejection, abuse, heartbreaks, career upheavals and betrayal. The beauty is that I trust the inner warrior that brings me back to that inner MANTLE that I was created to be.

This time and age need warriors that are trained to get back to that inner space, to operate based on love, humility and determination.

In the fear and disorder currently going on in the world, we need to remember that we are part of a natural selection and connected through love, and it's expression is the infinite light that we dare to shine on ourselves and others no matter what.

So dear reader, be brave now and rise above.

Like The lighted MANTLE, be a warrior and lead your life with wisdom and love.

I encourage you to walk with courage and determination, the path to your highest being and quintessence.

Always remember where you have been, where you come from and where you are going. You can only get better if you have faith and believe.

"IF I CAN DO IT, YOU CAN. IT'S POSSIBLE."

You are the UNSTOPPABLE MANTLE

You have all it takes to win.

I am a STAR born out of Scars.

Thank you.

YVONNE MUNDIH

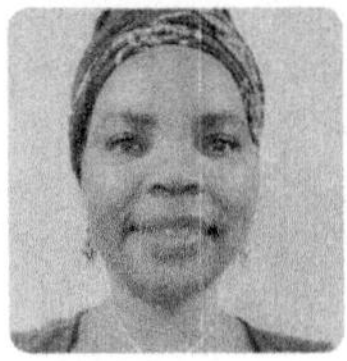

Best-selling author, speaker, coach, and educator, Yvonne is the founder of Building Hopes & Dreams Global LLC.

Yvonne uses her supports and empowers, to transform victims of domestic abuse and rejection to understand that no matter what storms come their way, they can thrive and not just survive.

Yvonne's passion is to empower and elevate the voices of women and children to understand that they are worthy.

Yvonne's mission is to build Mastermind schools around the world to teach and transform the lives of children between the ages of 3 and 25.

Yvonne has a degree's in African American Literature and Performing Arts and Mental Health Drug and Alcohol Counseling. A proud graduate from The Les Brown Power Voice Academy, Yvonne is speaking in March 2022 at The Women Leadership and Wellness International Expo in France.

"Am grateful to still be alive. The Spirit of my Grandmother lives within me."

https://linktr.ee/bhdglobal

8
CLAUDIA SPAHR
I LEFT FOR THE SAKE OF THE CHILDREN

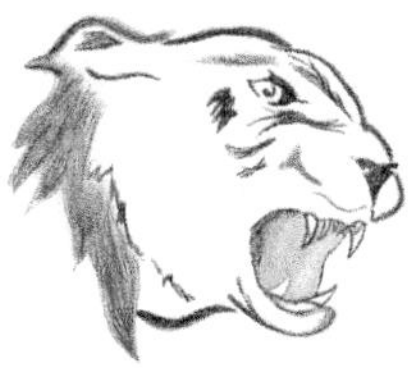

KICKED OUT

I'm looking in through the window of my home. It's early December and the Christmas tree has just been put up. It's decorated with different coloured baubles I found in a designer shop. There are other trinkets hanging on the tree, which the children helped me collect over the years. They've also carefully propped up snowy landscape cards we found at a market, while visiting my family in Switzerland. The living room is quiet and empty, just a few toys scattered here and there. It looks like a warm and loving space. Every item tells a story and there are happy memories of days spent drawing on the floor and dressing up and dancing with the kids. It's the living room of the house that I have known to be my home for the past seven years.

But I am shut out. The locks have been changed and my key doesn't fit. I'm hungrily looking through the window at the Yuletide festivities, like a street urchin from a Dickens tale. A court order has granted my ex full care of the children and exclusive access to the home. I only have a few hours to pack up my personal belongings and leave.

What kind of mother loses custody of her six, eight and eleven year-old? What did she do to deserve it? She must have done something wrong?

Let's just sit with that for a moment. We're going to explore our biases here.

Rewind to two years before the above scene. It was January 2018 when my husband filed for divorce because he was paranoid I would take the children and leave him. He never shared this with me, or the therapist we were seeing, because as a man brought up in a patriarchal society, he wasn't taught to express his fears or vulnerable feelings. He was conditioned to vanquish any threat that stood in the way of his power to control things. His lawyer and he had put together a suggestion for me: Their idea of a good deal[1] was: I sign over child custody and in return, I can stay living in the house with the family. Failure to sign would lead to court. Little did I know that refusing to enter into this medieval slave contract would lead to things getting much worse.

Most women experiencing coercive control or domestic violence know in their guts that the abuse is going to get worse, if they leave. And in my case, it did. It intensified. Leaving a partner with abandonment issues drives a dagger deeper into the core wound that most needs healing and the abuse can spiral out of control. There's even a term for it: Post-separation abuse. It's the reason why so many of us stay in abusive, co-dependent relationships and marriages, even when we know that the situation is harming us and the children.

Leaving is actually the most dangerous thing to do[2]. But it was the only thing I could do to protect the children.

For years I stayed for the children. Until I realised I had to leave for the children. If I couldn't keep myself safe, how on earth could I keep them safe? I remember messaging my mother after an argument with my husband that left me feeling particularly battered, denigrated, trivialised, and silenced.

"I have to save myself first. I'm no good to anyone in this state."

Of course, he read the text to my mother. He went into my phone behind my back. I'd lowered my standards on that years earlier. After all, I had nothing to hide. There was nothing to fuel his jealousy or his sporadic outbursts of rage. It was so easy to groom me into being loyal. I had recently quit my career as a foreign correspondent and was doing all I could to squeeze myself into the 'good wife' box. However, no matter what I did there was always something wrong. The toothpaste I'd bought was too expensive. The food I'd cooked was rubbish, and when it was good there wasn't enough of it. I'd birthed three children within the space of five years and was building a business from my laptop, while they were sleeping. No wonder I was exhausted at night when he felt entitled to my body. It was like our home was riddled with landmines that could go off any minute and each step required meticulous risk analysis. What I wanted most was to keep the peace and avoid any uncomfortable conversations that could spark his temper. We had to stay together for the children. I didn't want my children to come from a broken home. They deserved better.

In a last-ditch attempt at saving our marriage, I insisted on couples therapy, hoping it would fix our problems. After a few sessions, where the therapist wanted to see me mainly on my own, she advised me to 'get myself a good lawyer' and that she couldn't help us further. I didn't act on her advice. I'd probably still be thinking about contacting a lawyer, had he not filed for divorce.

Court proceedings turned into a nightmare, as we became entwined with a system that is coercive by nature. We were exposed to lawyers' agendas, judges' biases, and police failure to protect. Equally flawed were the government child protection agencies who were given an hour with each of us, in order to make assumptions that were open to interpretation by lawyers and judges. It all led to further entrapment.

I've come to see that the judiciary failed to grasp the bigger picture and what was actually going on in our family unit. Family Court became unsafe because abuse was being perpetuated by this very system[3].

Fear festers in an unsafe environment. Love thrives in a safe environment. It is that simple.

I know this not only from my experience of twelve years inside an unsafe marriage and the abuse I experienced through the courts but also from my work with women and children.

SAFE SPACES FOR WOMEN AND CHILDREN

It's time to introduce myself more formally:

Everything I do in my work is dedicated to providing safe spaces for women and children to thrive in. For 15 years I've been successful in the retreat and wellness world, curating transformational spaces for healing. Since 2013 - when I became pregnant with my daughter - I decided to focus solely on mothers and their children - society's most vulnerable and those who, I firmly believe, need this kind of nurturing more than anyone. Positive transformation can be most easily facilitated in a safe, non-competitive and loving space. It enables those present to connect with each other and their own repressed feelings, pent-up frustrations, challenges due to the expectations of motherhood, as well as their own wisdom and shared joyful experiences. We can only address trauma in a safe environment. As the days on retreat progress, the mums relax and begin supporting each other. As women, we feel sisterhood in our bones, like it is ´normal' or 'the way it should be'. In mainstream reality, it is harder to get into this mystical, ecstatic state. What I witness regularly on my retreats is an unlearning of our patriarchal ways and the remembering of a more loving, embodied, community-based way of being.

HOW PATRIARCHY HAS TAINTED US ALL

Our patriarchal systems have socialised us into hierarchies and pecking orders where the one on top controls. It is a 'power over' system, rather than 'power with'. A hierarchical system, based on a ruling top figure - usually a male God - relies on a culture of fear and punishment. This makes everyone feel unsafe, especially those being oppressed. Ironically those at the top aren't safe either because they're afraid of being toppled. It's an unnatural and unsustainable way to organise society in an interconnected world where everything affects everything else. What many of us have learnt growing up is that the stronger one wins, rather than resolving conflict through dialogue and mutual understanding.

For the mechanics of oppression to work people have to be isolated. That's how cults brainwash their members, by separating them from the outside world. Oppression ceases to have an impact when people think independently, take responsibility, and unite with a common goal. That's why when I bring mothers and children together on retreat the healing and transformation work is so easy. Coming together is the most subversive and powerful thing we can do.

HUMANITY HASN'T ALWAYS BEEN THIS OUT OF BALANCE

From Palaeolithic hunter-gatherer times through the advent of agriculture, women were revered and honoured as representatives of the mystery of the Divine Feminine. Out of the Goddess came life. When Semitic nomadic desert tribes invaded Canaan, the Goddess ("the abomination") was suppressed and erased[4]. The Abrahamic religions, Judaism, Christianity and Islam, shaped western culture by placing man over woman, and above nature. This patriarchal way of ruling led to the balance between feminine and masculine, between nature and humans, being lost. Power was taken by institutions, like the church, to decide on who gets to procreate with whom.

We are finally identifying the shortcomings and flaws of this dominator culture and how it has been the driving force behind colonialism, imperialism and white supremacy. We know there is a more balanced way of leading, in right relationship to the land and each other: Women, indigenous leaders, minorities and our youth all need seats at the tables where decisions are made.

BREAKING THE CHAIN OF PAIN

Our dominator framework has imbued everything because it controls how we think. It's a narrative we accept as normal. That's why we're blind to it. It's like fish in the sea not realising where they are. The ocean is the only thing they know.

Domination is a corner stone of coercive of control, of emotional abuse. It is insidious and complex[5]. And it is invisible: To the victim, the perpetrator and the system. That's why all the lawyers I've consulted with have told me that mentioning coercive control in a family courtroom will fall on deaf ears.

I remember years ago speaking out at a lunch with my in-laws. My ex was in a rage, trying to control where our toddler sat and what he was allowed to eat. I decided to share that he had physically abused me and that I was scared. When we are taught by the patriarchy to distrust the voice of a woman, it becomes acceptable to dismiss her and call her a liar. His father's response was denial and that, "No one in this family is a wife-beater." The response from his mother was, "He's always had a bad temper but he will calm down over time. Just wait until he gets older."

This is how we enable abuse from generation to generation, by mollycoddling our sons and silencing or blaming our daughters. But a woman isn't responsible for a man's feelings of rejection, inadequacy and alienation.

"You made me do it," is an accusation straight from the perpetrator's handbook.

My ex-mother-in-law also told me to bite my tongue. She suggested I leave the room when he lost his temper. It was the way she'd been taught to put up with misogyny. She had her own trauma to deal with and that was her coping mechanism.

But I was not willing to shut up nor be shut down. I was not willing to accept gas-lighting and projection as normal, until my body got sick from absorbing so much unrelenting injustice.

We're living in a traumatised world. Many of us have experienced some form of abuse or trauma[6]. We have to find a way to stop this.

GENERATIONAL HEALING

When I received the verdict that I had just lost parental care of my children on that dreary early December day in 2019, I was driving. Not the best place to receive a life-altering and damning sentence.

After two years of abusive litigation, which included delayed appeals, farcical trials and surreal court appearances, my ex was given a 'slap on the back and the fat cigar'. The courts favoured him on all counts and stripped me of everything. On top of exclusive access to the house, he was to receive monthly maintenance fees from me. In return, I would be able to see my children only four hours on a Wednesday, plus two Fridays and two Saturdays a month. I had just spent ridiculous amounts of money on legal fees on a malfunctioning system that was rigged against me from the get-go.

My immediate response was to scream. That is what my body needed to do. It was a scream that became a howling roar. Bloodcurdling, bone-chilling, and piercing, connecting me to other lifetimes, ancestors, the plight of women and the injustice of it all. I was being tortured inhumanely and my children were being forced to watch me being burnt alive. It was the roar of the wild woman, evoking those who have been silenced, ridiculed and maimed for speaking up. The roar of Feminine Mystery is the most primal of all. The Great

Unknown is part of the truth of who we are and what the patriarchy has been trying to shut down for millennia.

It wasn't so long ago that women were still being burned at stake for 'heresy'. In Spain - the country where this story takes place - The Inquisition was officially abolished only in 1834[7]. Two hundred years isn't a long time in a system that's been wreaking havoc for thousands of years. It's only two to three lifetimes, or seven generations. We know from epigenetic studies that trauma is passed from one generation to the next. We're basically healing lifetimes of control and domination.

To change a system that has been so violent towards women and children we need a paradigm shift. Masculine power is institutionalised and we see it played out in every aspect of our lives. We need those controlling the systems to acknowledge they are flawed and enable those with solutions and alternatives to join the discussion as equals. We need equity, inclusion, and diversity. We need a more right-brained, holistic approach to understand how it all interconnects, rather than isolating the individual parts, which is very left-brained. Then we need rehabilitation programmes, trauma recovery retreats and behaviour change incentives for the perpetrators of abuse. There simply aren't enough programmes for this demographic anywhere.

WHAT WOULD I SAY TO MY YOUNGER SELF?

Sometimes I think back to the moment at that window when I looked in at the Christmas tree. My Higher Self would say it was a moment of truth. It was like I was suspended in a void where I saw my whole life spread out before me, forwards and backwards through all time and space.

This twist of fate would push me to learn hard lessons. It would challenge me to lean into my compassion, raise the bar on my leadership, and become an even fiercer advocate for women and children. It would test my resilience, patience, and personal power, like nothing else.

I made the difficult decision to step away from my marriage, knowing it meant leaving my children in the hands of a man and his tribe who are refusing to look at their own trauma and patterns of coercive control. I am known as HolyMama - a curator of safe spaces for women and children, but I couldn't even keep my own children safe. Life is often like that: Your biggest challenge is your greatest gift to the world.

It boils down to this: I had to mother myself first and foremost. I had to find the oxygen mask in the debris before I could put it on. I had to face myself in the mirror and admit that I was in a coercive relationship that was breaking me. I had let him define what was acceptable behaviour and lost sight of my own values and beliefs.

There was another key moment when I realised just how bad the situation had gotten. It was when the police showed up outside our home during the interim sentence when we had shared custody in the 'nest house', where the children lived. Changeovers were riddled with drama. We were a textbook example of post-separation abuse.

My ex had just stolen my phone because he thought it contained evidence and he'd pushed me so hard onto the ground I had bruises. I wasn't going to press charges but neighbours called the police. I remember the police officer telling me to go to the hospital to show the bruises. "Women like you end up on the news,"[8] was the stark warning he gave me. I was biased in my belief that this only happened to women in trailer homes; not educated, financially independent, middle-class women like me.

By disentangling myself from codependent suffering that was toxic to all of us, I may have opened a door for healing for the whole family system. It might sound like the opposite happened because it did get so much worse first. What I do know from my work with healing is that there is a breaking down before there is a breakthrough. I need to trust that process.

If I hadn't stepped away I wouldn't have been able to see the patterns or make clear the invisible. I wouldn't have been able to stop the harsh words spoken to a mother by a father, and the pathetic defensive responses by a woman who had lost her own sense of dignity. I would have held back on becoming who I am today: An award-winning holistic business owner and multiple bestselling author and international speaker.

You cannot unshackle from entrapment until you understand how you have been colonised and controlled by a system, a society, group, partner or even parent. For me, leaving my marriage was my initiation into empathy for a traumatised world. I've seen that the depth of my suffering can be directly related to my highest potential, when I transform my pain into something greater than myself. That is what I chose and I would choose it time and time again.

I'd also tell my younger self this:

"Don't be ashamed of your feelings. Don't blame yourself. His humiliated fury is never justified, no matter what you did or said. It is never OK to shame, gaslight or make false allegations against someone, and walking on eggshells isn't a normal or acceptable way to live. You're an amazing mother and you definitely haven't failed your children by following your purpose in life, because it makes you a happier person. Keep your friends, they will show up for you when you need them. Never let anyone isolate or entrap you. Stick up for yourself because bullies are cowards at the end of the day. Don't cave in to demands or tricks. Stand in your own power. Connect with your heart. Raise your standards and clarify your boundaries. Learn to speak so articulately that even those who shut you down will hear you. Don't put other people's happiness before your own because you think you're not enough. Put yourself at the centre and then work from there. Real power comes from the centre."

WHAT WOULD I SAY TO MY CHILDREN

"I love you unconditionally and am here for you, whenever you need me. I know you think it's all my fault and that your father says I changed. I understand your loyalty towards your father and his family. I will do my best to not speak badly of them. Please understand that sometimes it's hard to do that while wanting to protect you at the same time. You might not always agree with my version of things. We all have different perspectives. My hope is that through our separation we will somehow become more whole. We all got hurt badly. I'm sorry you were misused by a system that was meant to decide for your best interests. It's not up to you to fix the mess the adults made. I'm doing what I can to ease your pain. I also realise that it's not my role as your mother to prevent suffering in a world that can be so cruel. What I can do is share what I learnt and how I got through it. My aim is to enable you with the wisdom and tools to navigate hard times and show you that kindness trumps all. I had to leave your father to find that strength within myself, so I could be strong for you. I know you don't like it that I wrote about us and I hope you can understand why I had to be a part of this book. I did it for wider mothering and for the children that aren't my own. Would it make you feel better if your story can prevent this from happening to another child?

And please know that I didn't leave because of my lack of love for you. I left because my love for you is greater than anything I have ever known. And I will always, always be your mother. No matter what.You grew inside my body and with each of your births I came close to death, to give you life. Sometimes I tell myself my most important mothering took place in those early years and when you were inside my womb. When you were part of me and I was part of you. When we were one."

Lawyers have advised me to refrain from being part of this book. However, as this chapter demonstrates, lawyers have failed me and my children and I will not be silenced. I decided to publish my story because it is time to bring the shame around abuse to light. This conversation enables others to talk about it and leave an unhealthy relationship, so that they too can thrive in life.

Stories can change someone's life because give others permission to talk about it.

---

1. "Abusive fathers are more than twice as likely to petition for sole custody of their children as non-abusive fathers." Mary Przekop in the Seattle Journal of Social Justice. One More Battleground: Domestic Violence, Child Custody, and the Batterers' Relentless Pursuit of their Victims Through the Courts
2. "It's become a well-known saying that 'leaving is the most dangerous time.' We know it's dangerous, because more than half of men who kill their intimate partners do so either after they leave, or indicate they're about to. Victim survivors know that leaving is the most dangerous time, because they know how much the perpetrator needs to be in control. https://www.vwt.org.au/thetrap/, Episode Four
3. "Litigation involving child support and custody is one of the most common ways domestic- violence perpetrators prolong contact with their victims, not only is the abuser finding a new avenue for harassment, but he's also telling his victim that the court isn't a safe place for her." T. K. Logan, behavioural scientist and professor, University of Kentucky
4. Archaeological remains from Palaeolithic and Neolithic times show that there was a deep honour for the Feminine, for fertility and the earth. There is no evidence of any weapons from this era, implying there was no violence or wars. Safety and peace were prevalent. Works by Marija Gimbutas and Joseph Campbell, Mysteries of the Feminine Divine
5. Amnesty International identified in 1973 the 'universal tools of torture and coercion'. Experts agree that these same principles of psychological abuse are used by perpetrators of domestic abuse. Coercive control or 'thought reform' indoctrinates the minds of those subjected to it
6. The World Health Organization estimates that 30 per cent of women worldwide will experience physical or sexual violence in the context of an intimate relationship. This means that a similar percentage of men are perpetrators of violence.
7. The Tribunal of the Holy Office of the Inquisition, also called Spanish Inquisition, was one of the most violent and coercive judicial institutions to combat heresy. Its brutal methods led to widespread death and suffering.
8. More than half of women and girls killed by men are murdered by their current or previous partners. Femicide Watch Report, UN

CLAUDIA SPAHR

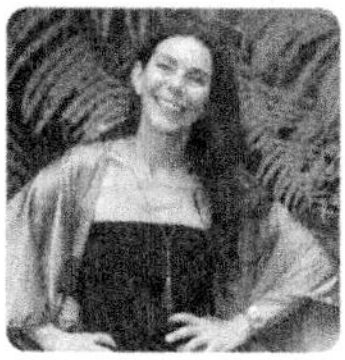

Claudia Spahr curates safe spaces for women and children. She founded HolyMama in 2013, with the birth of her daughter. Claudia has trained retreat leaders in over 20 countries, across 6 continents, and she's hosted hundreds of transformational retreats around the world. Having had three children in her forties Claudia wrote a book about later motherhood, which became an international bestseller and was published in 6 languages, including Chinese and Korean. Claudia is a keynote speaker and feminine leadership mentor and has won a Best Women in Business Award for her international achievements. Before becoming a health and wellness pioneer she worked over a decade in the media as a radio broadcast journalist and TV foreign correspondent.

Find more information about Claudia's books, retreats, online programmes and leadership trainings at http://holymama.info/ and http://claudiaspahr.com/
Invite her to speak: claudia@holymama.info
Social media www.instagram.com/_holymama_/

9

MICHELLE EL-DIN

UNSTOPPABLE

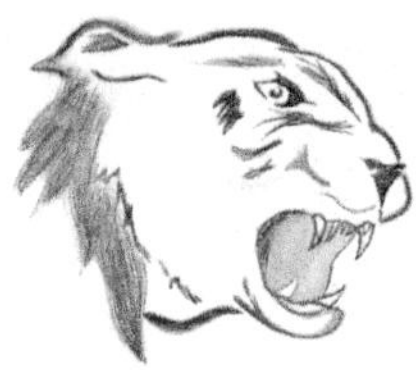

---

*Please note that all names have been changed to protect the identity of the individuals involved.

INTRODUCTION:

I distinctly remember the little boy asking his mum, "Mummy, why has that lady got blood all over her face?"

I was sitting in the waiting room in the A and E department of our local hospital after *James had hit me over the head with a hammer when I'd asked for his help to put together a chest of drawers. James had called an ambulance and then fled the house.

I lied to the doctor about what had happened. I said that I'd been doing some DIY and accidentally tripped and banged my head on the corner of the drawers. The doctor didn't question me and looked at the cut on my head, checked that I wasn't suffering from concussion and then sent me on my way.

Walking home from the hospital alone was when reality hit me, I realised that I could have lost my life that morning, and I decided that it was to be the final incident.

On my return to the house that I shared with James and two other friends, I picked up the phone and confided in a good friend who then came around. I told her what had been happening and she encouraged me to report everything to the police as I still had bruises on my face for evidence. Part of me didn't want to as I didn't have the strength to go through any questioning or more emotional distress by recalling everything; I just felt like curling up. However, I knew in order to protect myself that I had to, and deep down I knew this had to stop.

It was nearly two years after the first incident that I took that step, however, I am so glad I did. My world is now a million miles away from the world that I thought my ex had created for me, and I am no longer the shell of a person that I was after leaving the relationship.

Leaving was one of the hardest things that I've had to do, however, I have gone from rock bottom to become an unstoppable, confident and successful businesswoman and mum, leading a life that I choose, and I'd like to share my story to empower you to do the same.

WHERE IT ALL BEGAN:

I met James at the local sports centre where he worked as a gym instructor. When I first saw him, I thought nothing of him. He certainly wasn't my usual, tall, dark and handsome type. He was always friendly though and we got chatting. After seeing him on a few occasions I agreed to go for a drink with him.

Over the following weeks, we spent more time together and eventually became a couple. This was the start of nearly two years of hell.

After about nine months of being together, I moved into the house that James rented with two male friends. I don't remember how far into our time cohabiting that the first incident occurred, however, I do remember that in no way did I think that it would be one of many occasions that I would be physically abused by my partner.

All of the incidents occurred in our house. I would often wonder how our housemates didn't notice my bruises and black eyes. Although I became very good at wearing makeup in the right way, coming up with excuses and I would also hide in our bedroom pretending that I had other things to do or that I was ill. I'm sure everyone thought that I was unsociable, which I hated, but I thought better that, than to have to explain my injuries. James carried on his life as normal as if what he did didn't matter. This made me feel worthless and my self-esteem really plummeted.

I used to ask James why he hit me, and he would say that he just saw 'red mist' and that he couldn't control his actions. He always apologised and sometimes even cried, stating that it would never happen again. Me being the empathetic person that I am, actually felt sorry for him. I think I even said that it was ok and for him not to worry?!

Most incidents occurred after an argument. One Valentine's Day I had sent some flowers to James' place of work. Being a bit of an old romantic, I thought that I was doing something nice and a bit different, but he didn't see it that way. When he got home, he went upstairs to get changed so I put the flowers in a vase on the side. He came downstairs and was fuming; asking me why I'd embarrassed him in front of his work colleagues. I apologised and said I was just trying to do something nice and that I was sorry if I'd upset him. He hit me and smashed the vase of flowers on the lounge floor. I then tried to get up off the floor where I'd landed when he hit me, but he grabbed me by my hair and tried to drag me over the broken glass. My jumper rode up my back as he dragged me, and the glass cut my back drawing blood. I cried and said to him that I needed to get away and that I was going to phone my parents. I tried to get up to grab the house phone, but he pushed me down again and took the phone from the side and smashed it under his foot on the floor. I felt scared and alone and I knew that our housemates wouldn't be back until later that evening as they both worked late shifts. Once I'd recovered from the shock and the fact that I would be unable to get help, my thoughts turned to cleaning the blood-stained carpet so no one would know what had happened (goodness knows why!). I cleaned up and then went upstairs to sit in the bedroom and cried uncontrollably while James remained downstairs playing on the computer as if nothing had happened. I felt alone and unsure of what to do. I was too scared to call anyone on my mobile and also ashamed that this was happening to me.

I carried on my life as best I could, hiding my bruises and black eyes as much as possible, however, as more incidents occurred, I began to lose myself. I stopped seeing my family and friends regularly. Prior to being with James, I was known for having a really busy social life. However, I didn't want to admit to anyone what I was going through so I used to come up with excuses to not see people and no one ever questioned me as I would often say that I was busy meeting other friends.

Eventually, I lost my job due to the vast amount of time off I'd had. I often couldn't face going into work because my self-esteem and confidence were at rock bottom and sometimes I couldn't even face going outside. I began to slip into a deep depression. I'd stay in bed for long periods of time, and I was constantly drained. I avoided our housemates as much as I could. Despite them being really lovely guys, I just wasn't comfortable explaining my injuries to them and I didn't want to be questioned.

One summer James stamped on my foot so hard, following an argument that I thought he had broken it. I couldn't face going to the hospital, so I carried on with a severely bruised and swollen foot. Due to it being summer I continued to wear sandals because I thought that no one would notice my feet and told anyone that questioned me that we'd been bowling, and I'd accidentally dropped a bowling ball on my foot.

On another occasion, we visited my parents when I had a black eye. I tried to cover up the bruise as much as I could with make-up, and James and I had already planned our excuse before arriving. We agreed that we would say that we had been playing tennis, which wasn't unusual given that it was summer and that we both enjoyed playing, and that the ball had accidentally hit my eye, hence the bruising. My parents didn't question it and sadly I found it easier to lie to people close to me because I didn't want to hurt them with the truth.

James used to play football most Sunday mornings. One particular Sunday he returned from football with a friend. He'd left his phone in our bedroom on the side while he was in the bathroom. Something drew me to his phone to take a look, so I did, and my heart sank. I found messages saying 'thanks for our steaming session' from a girl called *Jodie. I had no idea who Jodie was or that James had been going to the gym with her. James went downstairs and I was still in the bedroom, again hiding myself away because I had a black eye. When he finally came upstairs, I confronted him and asked him who this girl was and what she meant by 'steamy session'. He started shouting saying that I shouldn't have been looking at his phone and punched me in the face. I said that I'd had enough, and I was leaving. He then slammed the bedroom door shut and got out his karate belt from the wardrobe (he went to karate classes) and said that if I left or told anyone then he would hang himself. He then proceeded to put the belt around his neck and tried to hang himself from the bedroom door. My natural instinct was to try and stop him, which I did. I felt panicked and had no idea what to do. James started to cry, and I told him not to be silly and that everything would be ok. As always, I was apologising and sympathising with him; I have no idea why I did this! Of course, I didn't want him to end his life, but on reflection, he had no right to have my sympathy after all he had put me through. After

James had calmed down, he went downstairs and went out with his friend, and I was left alone in the house dealing with the consequences and my thoughts around what he had done.

After every incident, James would always either leave the house or leave me alone in our bedroom which left me feeling isolated, numb and not knowing what to do. I can honestly say that these were some of the darkest days of my life.

Throughout all of this James had managed to make me believe that the abuse was my fault and if it wasn't for my actions then he would not have hurt me as I was always the one that started the arguments by questioning his disrespectful behaviour.

HOW DO I MOVE FORWARD?

After the final incident described at the start of this chapter, I went to the police station and then returned to my parent's house. I had mixed emotions. I felt depressed, worthless, anxious, scared and ashamed by what had happened. There was also still an emotional attachment to James despite what he had done. Although I knew that I would never be with him again, and I didn't want to be, there was still a sense of sadness around the whole situation.

I also felt dreadfully guilty knowing that I had lied to my parents for so long and that the whole situation must've hurt them so badly. Being a parent now myself, I can only imagine what that must've felt like for them.

I remember feeling like damaged goods and completely empty inside not knowing how to move forward, and yet I mustered the strength to do so. I knew that there was only one way up from rock bottom.

HOW IT ALL CHANGED:

Rebuilding myself wasn't an easy journey; it was really hard some days. However, with time, I began to feel like myself again. I now feel unstoppable, and I hope that this section of the chapter will help you work towards that too.

There are no timescales or deadlines as to how long it takes to heal. Don't pressurise yourself, however, appreciate that it is part of the journey to regaining your wonderful self.

HERE ARE FOUR THINGS THAT I WANT TO SHARE WITH YOU THAT HELPED ME TO ACCEPT WHAT HAPPENED AND MOVE FORWARD POSITIVELY:

1. **Accepting that toxic people will never change, they will only change you:**

It's easy to believe them when they say, "It won't happen again", "I'm so sorry, I don't mean to", however, once is enough. Look at their actions, not just their words.

Unfortunately, they will never change, and abusive behaviour is not ok; there is no excuse for it, and you are not responsible for their actions. It's certainly not your job to try and make them change. Do not feel sorry for them in any way; it's you that is suffering and losing yourself and it's not your fault.

2. **Step away from the stigma that you're weak:**

There is sometimes a stigma attached to victims of domestic abuse that they're weak. However, it is in fact the perpetrators that are weak as they have to control and belittle someone else to gain their 'power' to make up for their own insecurities.

During and after trauma, it is easy to feel vulnerable and that there are challenges everywhere. The path forward can appear very daunting and scary. I remember being worried about what people would think of me for having stayed in an abusive relationship for so long. However, when I finally had the confidence to open up, everyone around me was supportive and no one judged me.

Remember, you are not what's happening to you, and you're not weak or broken. Abusers are very good at making their victims feel like it's their fault. Don't be ashamed of what's happened to you; there is nothing wrong with you; normal human beings don't go around hurting other people.

I've learnt that I was definitely not to blame and some of the strongest people I know have an abusive past.

3. **Remember your worth:**

Never forget who you are, what you believe in and who you were before this relationship.

Recall the morals and values that you hold. Remember that you deserve respect at ALL times and never lose sight of your boundaries.

You can't control how other people act; however, you can choose how you react to them. Believe in you, and your ability; we all have so much to offer the world. Reach out to family/a friend, a support organisation—take that first step knowing that you are worth a million times more.

If you don't respect or value yourself, then no one else will. You may be at rock bottom now, but this experience will help to shape you into a stronger human being. We all have a strength within us that we're often unaware of until we have to use it.

I would highly recommend the book 'I'm Worth More' by Rob Moore which will help you realise your real value.

Know your worth and never value yourself on someone else's inability to do so.

4. **Finally, practice gratitude daily:**

This helped me immensely on my journey to heal. Every night think of three things for which you're grateful. It can be something small such as managing to get out of bed that day, a chat with a friend, a cup of tea, a hot shower or a lovely walk.

This daily practice will switch your mindset to become more positive and within weeks it will help you to appreciate the little things in life and you will take comfort in such things.

CONCLUSION:

When you're feeling at rock bottom and considering whether life is worth living or not, it's hard to find the strength and purpose to want to carry on. However, bravery comes from looking yourself in the eye and believing in you and how your past will help to shape you. You can and will feel whole again when you give attention and time to healing and investing in yourself. If I can, then anyone can.

I want to end the chapter with a poem called 'Unstoppable' by John Mark Green. May it give you the strength and belief to know that you are truly unstoppable, that your past doesn't determine your future and you hold the power to command more from your life.

UNSTOPPABLE:

You tried to cage her and contain her, drain her of her worth,

beat her down to nothing, with relentless fists of words,

tried to control and de-soul her, but she is resilient,

bamboo to your storm, bending but not breaking,

now taking back her true form.

Courage building like a tsunami, ready to lay waste,

to your city of empty promises.

She will rise above your shallow ruins like the moon in all her fullness;

free and beautiful, so luminous.

Your hungry night tried to devour her, but she made her own light which darkness could not swallow.

You are hollow and aimless, but she carries life hidden within;

a seedling growing skyward toward the sun of better things.

Your heart is salted earth, and your body a walking mausoleum.

You love control and fear freedom,

mistaking intimidation for true power, and captivity for devotion.

Devoid of emotion

you're dead inside,

and you wanted to bury her with you in a graveyard of lies.

But she will rise. She will shine. She will.

She is so much more powerful than you.

Unstoppable.

-John Mark Green

MICHELLE EL-DIN

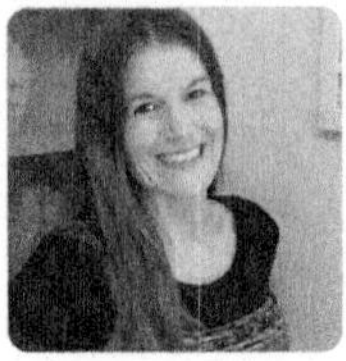

Michelle is a single mum and a business owner of a successful sales Recruitment Agency which has been voted 'Sales Recruitment Agency of the Year-UK' for three consecutive years. Her company was awarded 'Top 30 Fastest-Growing Private Companies to Watch in 2021'.

Michelle is a Business Master for Jessica Cunningham's: Conscious Female Entrepreneurs business venture. (Jessica starred in UK tv show The Apprentice.)

Since experiencing a domestic abusive relationship, Michelle has regained her strength and then some. She has successfully rebuilt her life from rock bottom and is passionate about empowering others to do the same, helping them find their true calling by removing the limiting beliefs that are preventing them from moving forward and living their best life.

You can contact Michelle by emailing her at:
Michelle@kmerecruitment.com
or by connecting with her on
Linkedin: https://www.linkedin.com/in/michelle-el-din-54248132/

10

CHRIS WILLIAMS

OUR STORY ISN'T OVER. WE GET TO WRITE THE ENDING

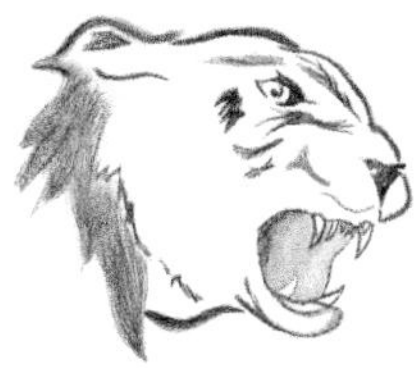

SNOW GLOBE EFFECT

The snow globe, an item that makes us think of winter, a childhood trinket, and a gift-shop staple. It is an object that evokes holiday cheer. We shake it and watch the snow peacefully fall to the bottom of the globe and for just a moment, we are at peace.

During a conversation with a woman who had courageously agreed to be a guest on my podcast, to share her Domestic Abuse story, she described her experience as being in a snow globe. It felt like someone had shaken her world upside down as she lived in a chaotic relationship. That description has stayed with me since our discussion as it was not one I had heard before when discussing the effects of abuse. I can see it in my mind so clearly, someone shaking the snow globe as you are being tossed around not knowing where you will land once the "shaking" stops.

Domestic Abuse, two words that I had not heard when I was growing up. The emotional, psychological, and physical abuse that I suffered and watched in my childhood was my normal. I didn't know there was a name for it until I learned more about it as an adult, after many unhealthy relationships and two abusive marriages. I didn't understand why I kept getting involved with the same type of men, one's with narcissistic personalities. I didn't know there was help available to leave an abusive relationship. I didn't understand why men who said they loved me, could hurt me so badly emotionally and physically.

I Was Told Not to Tell

I was that girl who wanted so desperately to be loved and escape the toxic environment I was living in. I dreamed of the "white knight" rescuing me, protecting me, taking care of me, and living happily ever after with the white picket fence, two children and a dog. I read romance novels and I watched Hallmark movies where the characters fell in love and had a beautiful life and family...that is what I dreamed for myself.

Instead, my reality was filled with the memories of my older brother's friends laying on top of me in my bedroom one summer day as they were experimenting with sex. I was told not to tell.

Instead, my reality was the beatings I endured from a wooden spoon, wooden board, belt, back of a hand wearing big gold rings smacked across my face or a chair being thrown across the room breaking the drywall, as the anger erupted toward me. I tried to tell, but what went on behind closed doors, stayed behind closed doors.

Instead, my reality was the boy who raped me at age 13 as he whispered, "I love you." I was told not to tell as he was over 18.

Instead, my reality was the coach who told me daily he loved me, and I was "special" as he groomed me, and others, for years. I was told not to tell.

Instead, my reality was the man that I would meet at the end of my senior year of high school and marry at 22. He would be my first abusive marriage. I was begged not to tell.

I did tell but I was told he loved me and would go to Alcoholics Anonymous to get the help he needed, and I went to Al-Anon. Even when 911 was called by our neighbors after a particularly bad fight at our apartment. They heard me screaming for my life as he was sitting on top of me with a knife to my throat. The police arrived, but all they did was tell him to go to the hospital because it looked like he had broken his hand from hitting the wall. All this took place before we were even married, yet we still became husband and wife as I thought "if I loved him enough, he would change and stop drinking." I left a year later as I realized two things...1) one of us was going to end up being killed and I didn't want it to be me, or 2) he was going to kill someone while driving drunk and I couldn't live with myself if that ever happened.

Instead, my reality was the man who would become my second abusive marriage. The red flags were there from the beginning; however, I again ignored them and didn't walk away when I had the chance. The abuse was much more emotional and psychological... there were no bruises but there was verbal abuse, manipulation, emotional blackmail, gaslighting, lying, privacy invasion, character assassination, stalking, digital abuse and so much more. This marriage was much harder to leave as we had a child together.

It took me two attempts to leave this marriage. The average time it takes a woman to leave an abusive relationship is seven times. The first time I left, I had filed for divorce but a few weeks before the divorce was to be finalized, he was rushed to the hospital and was not expected to live as he had contracted "flesh-eating bacteria." His body was already shutting down by the time they got him into his first surgery. He had four surgeries in five days. He did survive and once released from the hospital, needed 24-hour at-home care for months after. Since we were still "legally married" and no family members offered to help, his co-workers packed up my belongings and my son and I moved back to our home and there I stayed for two more years. I made a plan for the second time to leave and this time when I left, I knew I would never return.

In 2015, after working with a life coach, selling my business and as another relationship was "on a break", I took a very well-deserved trip to Maui and invited my mom to come along. I was flipping through channels on the TV one afternoon while my mom was napping and there was an episode on the Steve Harvey Talk Show about vision boards.

Sitting on a beach on the shores of Maui is where Livin' the Visions was created. As I watched the sunset go down and began to write my dreams in my journal.

I began to visualize what I wanted my life to look like as I began to heal. I wanted to take the lessons that my life coach taught me and begin to understand how to use these "tools" to help women recover from abuse. I wanted to discover if there was help available for women who wanted to leave abusive relationships. I wanted to learn how to stop the generational cycle of abuse so that my son didn't repeat the same patterns I witnessed from my grandmother, my mother and me.

I got certified as a Life Coach with a focus on Domestic Violence Recovery and started Livin' the Visions to **Educate**, **Empower**, and help women **Envision** life without abuse. I also got certified as a DV Advocate.

EDUCATE

Education is key to healing. Learning the definition of abuse, the many types of abuse, the cycle of abuse, what type of men abuse, understanding the emotional, physical and symptoms of abuse are key to healing. Educating yourself on how abuse affects your family, your children, your friends, your job, and your self-identity are steps to healing. Learning that there is help and support before, during and after you have left the relationship, is part of healing. So many women say they didn't know help was available by calling a Domestic Abuse hotline where advocates are available 24 hours a day to talk to.

Understanding domestic abuse is a pattern of behaviors used to gain or maintain **POWER AND CONTROL** is healing. Learning the signs of unhealthy and healthy relationships is part of the healing journey. Identifying the red flags and knowing when to walk away is part of the journey. Using your voice to share your stories and help educate others on Domestic Abuse may save a life and is part of the healing journey.

EMPOWER

Empowering yourself is key to healing. Who are we without the abuse?

I like to use the example of the character Julia Roberts played Maggie Carpenter in the 1999 film Runaway Bride. Throughout the movie, Ike (Richard Gere) interviews Maggie's (Julia Roberts) former fiancés. These are men that she had left at the altar on their wedding day. One question he asked during these interviews was how Maggie liked her eggs cooked. The men would always respond with, "Scrambled, just like me" or "Poached, just like me." In every relationship, Maggie liked her eggs just like her partner did. Ike, talking about Maggie's past, said, "You were so lost, you didn't even know what kind of eggs you liked! With the priest, you wanted scrambled. With the deadhead, it was fried..." Maggie responded defensively, "That is called changing your mind." Ike replied, "**No, that's called not having a mind of your own.**"

Reclaiming your sense of self, your identity, creating your life path, your surroundings and flipping the script from victim to survivor mentality, is part of your healing journey. Reclaiming your power begins with your mental health. By speaking positive affirmations, repeating "I AM" statements, shifting your automatic negative thoughts, setting boundaries, learning your values, developing self-confidence, loving yourself, being grateful, asking for what you want, learning to not just have a voice but a powerful voice, letting go of fear and becoming courageous are all part of your next chapter.

ENVISION

Envisioning/Dreaming is key to healing. When you begin to heal, slowly you begin to dream again of the possibilities for your future.

The first dream I told everyone, after my second divorce in 2009, was that I wanted to open a spa where I would create an environment for women to relax, breathe, get pampered and escape from reality for a period of time.

In 2011, that dream became a reality, sort of. I opened Dolce Vita Hair & Nail Salon! I had no experience running a small business and had no knowledge of how to do hair or nails but that didn't stop me. How did this happen? The power of envisioning and talking to everyone about what my dreams were. The reason for this is 1) you never know who you are going to talk to who might know someone that can help you, and 2) the more you are speaking and visualizing your dreams the Reticular Activating System (RAS) in your brain starts to take in this information and processes it as being important to you. Your RAS is the thing that analyses what incoming information is relevant to you (and your survival) and lets only the most important stuff through – it actively blocks the rest of the info (so you are not aware of it). So, what you are putting to the Universe and what you are feeding your mind is what you are going to start seeing everywhere you look.

Here is how the story goes, I started telling everyone that this was my dream. I started meeting people who had owned similar types of businesses. I started going to spas to see how they were designed, what services they provided, what their prices were, what their websites and marketing looked like, and started searching to see what spa businesses were for sale. One day while I was lying on the bed next to my son as he was reading before bed, a voice in my head said go to Craigslist and look for spas for sale. Once my son fell asleep, I looked on Craigslist and the first business that was for sale was a salon in my neighborhood and was five minutes from my home which was perfect. I called and met with the owner and within 45 days of the first meeting, I had bought the business, signed a lease, remodeled, renamed, rebranded, and opened the doors to Dolce Vita Salon!

People thought I was crazy for my belief that visualizing could make "Shit" happen until they started seeing the life I was creating. It's not just cutting out photos and putting them on a vision board and waiting for those things to magically appear, there is a process to it, and you have to believe in the power of manifesting. As a Domestic Violence Recovery Coach and Personal Development Coach, I work with my clients on envisioning life without abuse and teaching them how to create the life they envision for themselves. It is work, it is belief, it is stepping into your courageous self, it is learning to ask for help and it is having faith in yourself that if you can dream it, you can achieve it.

Envisioning isn't just about material things; it's about how you want to live your life. Here is another example of how it works. I have done this exercise with clients, and I did it for myself when I was ready to date again. I made a list of all the things I wanted in a man. I wrote down every little detail, even down to the color of socks I wanted the man to wear. It would be impossible to get 100% of what you want out of a relationship, but it is a good way to discover what you will not tolerate and/or settle for moving forward. I will be married to the man I envisioned, for six years in January of 2022. And he planned the wedding which was just the two of us on a beach in Kauai!

When we became empty-nesters, I envisioned a condo on the water with a west-facing view to watch the sunsets...even down to the paint color I wanted on the walls. It took two years of manifesting, but in 2017, I bought that condo on the water.

In 2019, when COVID affected all our lives, we got serious about the boat we had been talking about. We went through the steps again of talking with everyone about boats, test driving boats, looking at boats, making a list of what we wanted on a boat, cutting out pictures of boats to put on our vision board, and taking our boating license classes so that we would be ready for when we found the boat. Three months after COVID shut everything down, we bought our first boat and that's how we managed our mental health during the COVID shutdown.

I know the stories make it sound simple, but creating the life that you envision is work, belief and understanding that you must be ready for those things that you create and envision in your life. The mind and Universe are powerful tools. Once you put things out to the Universe, you must be ready to receive them, or you could miss your opportunity.

One last story of creating your vision I'd like to share is one about my husband (well he was my boyfriend at the time). He was not the type that believed in the power of manifesting. His dream car was a Range Rover Sport. He talked about how much he loved this type of car and would love to own one someday. As he began to talk more about it, he kept seeing Range Rovers everywhere. (Hasn't that happened to you when you start thinking about something that you have passion around, you start seeing it everywhere?) One day in 2013, I asked him if he had ever driven a Range Rover, he answered "No." I replied, "then how do you know if a Range Rover is your dream car?" He did not have an answer. I suggested he drive one and said we were going to the dealership that weekend to do just that. Of course, he loved the test drive as they take you out back and let you drive over a designated course to show you all that the car can do. Now he was really infatuated with the car! I told him to cut out a picture of the color and type of Range Rover he wanted and add that to his vision board (as we each had our own) and hang the board next to his bed so he would see it every morning and evening. Six months later, he walked into my salon in the middle of the day with a big grin on his face as had he bought himself a used 2007 Range Rover. He still has that car today and loves it just as much as he did when he bought it.

Freedom

There are several definitions for the word Freedom. But for survivors of domestic abuse, it is difficult to feel true freedom even after we've left the abusive relationship. Creating our freedom can only be done without self-judgment, self-blame, and self-criticism. Freedom is realized when we are committed to falling in love with ourselves, to owning our story, and living our truth.

It had been a long road to Freedom in my story, but in 2019, that chapter of **Power & Control** had come to a close. As I sat outside a hotel 287 miles away from home, after reading the final decision from the arbitrator, I looked up and saw a flag flying above me in the wind with the light shining behind it. It was the biggest sign I could have received from the Universe. I shouted, "I'm Finally Free!"

They asked her,

"How do you know the healing is working?"

She answered,

"When your mind is no longer governed by the past and when you feel peace in situations where you use to feel tension. You more easily connect with joy and happily use boundaries to protect your well-being. The healing is real when your mind feels lighter and loving yourself becomes more natural."

— YUNG PUEBLO CLARITY & CONNECTION

I want to leave you with this one question, if your life were a book, how would you write your next chapter? Education is key to breaking the cycle of abuse. Healing from the abuse will help you write the next chapter of your story. Each of us are Survivors and sharing our stories can **Educate**, **Empower,** and help women **Envision** life without abuse.

Remember, our story isn't over, we get to write the ending.

CHRIS WILLIAMS

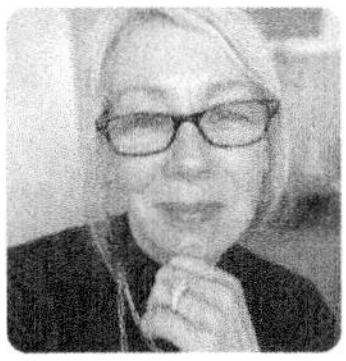

Chris Williams, Domestic Violence Recovery Coach, Personal Development Coach, Survivor of Domestic Violence, and host of *Livin' the Visions* podcast works with survivors of domestic violence to **Educate, Empower** and help women **Envision** life without abuse and reshape their life stories. She is passionate about her mission because as a Survivor, she believes when women personify a deep sense of self-love, self-acceptance, and self-belief, they become unstoppable and have the courage to Break the Cycle.

Chris focuses on 1:1 online and group coaching throughout the US. Her personal experiences allow Chris to create trust with her clients and assist them in creating life balance, identifying their strengths and values, overcoming fears and limiting beliefs, setting goals plus ongoing assistance in changing the script of automatic negative thoughts.

Chris, her husband and two adult boys, live in Washington State where she enjoys boating, horseback riding and many outdoor adventures.

Website: www.livinthevisions.com
Email: chris@livinthevisions.com
Instagram: @livinthevisions

11

BELLEE LV

YOU CAN HAVE IT ALL WITHOUT THE STRUGGLE, SUFFERING & PAIN

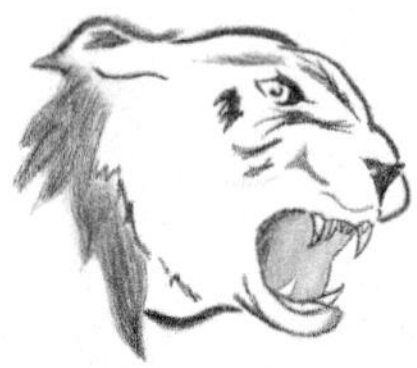

Like every other girl I always yearned for a happy family, a Complete family!

Have you heard of needing a man to keep a woman safe in the society?

Yes I needed a man, a father to protect my family! My father died when I was a year old. My timid and illiterate mother had no idea how to run his business and we lost our home and all the savings. She worked three jobs in a day to support us financially. I still remember how while waiting for her to finish her cleaning and housemaid job, I would be playing at one corner. I was always sticking with my mum until I turned four years old.

Mum sent me to my grandma's house and she continued working hard for the family. Grandma brought me up till I completed my kindergarten. Mum would visit me once a week. I was a mischievous girl in kindergarten! I was a bully then. There was once my classmate said 'eh girls cannot fight! Girls are weak!' I broke his leg!! Again and Again grandma got called to the principal's office. It was a weekly routine for her. Yet, she never gave up on me and until today she always believed in me.

I went back home when I was six years old, when My older sister finally got married. We were all happy for her. Finally a man in the family. To me, he was like a father figure. My sister was working three jobs in a day! Struggling to feed the family. Immediately after getting married, she was already pregnant! She worked all the way until she gave birth.

Once, my sister worked at night at a clinic. In the day,he was there chiding me, spoiling me and correcting me. And at night, with my sister at work he would enter my room and show his love by molesting me. I stayed silent. This was love from a man! The same man who showed me love is hurting me!

Meanwhile he began abusing all of us including my sister. My sister, my mother and I stayed silent. Our silence made him stronger. He continued entering my room until I turned 13, when I had my periods. And by then all I knew was that I have to give something to get love from men!

In school we were taught to call the police if there is violence at home! So many times I did! When the police arrived, my sister would pretend nothing happened

Each time, after every fight, after every abuse, they would sit down happily and act like nothing had happened!

All I understood by then was it's ok for men to abuse us, to do anything to us! That's love!

There was once when he hit my sister and literally split her head into two that we were galvanised to wake up and talk. To tell him to leave!! I decided to tell my sister what happened so that my niece won't go through what I did and suffer in silence like me!

My sister finally divorced him! He was no longer in our life. I spent my entire childhood feeling fear for myself and the women in the family! Thank god it was all over!

When I grew older, I looked for a man who would protect me. So I found myself a gangster who used his muscle to get his way. He was in and out of prison and all he did was build up massive debts. I was ok with that because that's all I knew about love! It's ok for the woman to work hard and support the man as long he loves her! So to me it was normal. Where was I? I was broken, torn, emotionally and verbally abused and tired of being pregnant. Ready to give it all up! I had no avenue in front of me. I had gone from one emotional prison to the other to visit him. I'd tied up and gagged up my own potential and created a victim of myself.

I realise struggle has been my identity! Always working hard and always feeling not deserving for all the things that come to my life.

I thought I had achieved success when I independently cleared the debt! And I was able to be both that man and woman for my daughter. I cherished that identity. I was really proud of it and then I realized that this is not what I want to live with, and this is definitely not the identity I want my daughter to carry! I want to live life to the fullest with compassion and love. To be able to forgive is the real indicator of love.

When my daughter was born, I filed for a divorce. I choose to not let her go through and be part of my victim story. I choose to protect her.

Being a single mum at age of 23, my ex-husband left me with $10,000 worth of debts, all under my name, when my daughter was three months old. He was back in prison and I was left to fend entirely for myself.

With my three-month-old in my arms, I worked three jobs a day, just like my mother and sister. I followed the same story and pattern without realising it. I was then also supporting two of my other family members. It was tough but struggling was in our blood It was normal to struggle.

I was working and struggling very hard for my daughter and family and that was my identity. I was working as a maid/helper in the morning, tutor in the moon and & debt management officer in the evening!

I realised that needed to change and that things were not going to work if I kept going the way I was going.

It was a chance ad on Facebook that changed it for me. I decided to heal myself, end the cycle and upgrade my consciousness. I was ready to do anything just to feed the family! I just wanted to change my life and clear my debts. I wanted to give my mum and my daughter a better life. Enough of struggling!

So I stepped out from working and enrolled myself in a personal development programme and graduated from a business entrepreneurship course!

I then took up a Beauty and Nutrition Natural Healing Course while holding my 18 months old. I travelled with my mum! My mum helped me to look after her while I was learning. Every four hours I had to stop to breastfeed her. When I came out of the hall, I would see them sitting down and waiting for me. It was at that time that I told myself I would do whatever it takes to give them the best life. After I graduated, I set up my own mobile spa and I worked hard. I cleared $10,000 debts in two months.

It was so tiring and frustrating. I left home in the morning when my daughter was sleeping and when I came home she was already asleep for the night too!

Nine years ago I suffered from a face stroke and I felt like the world had crashed in on me! I had self low esteem and low confidence! So when I decided to do business, my intention was to help as many women as possible to realise that being beautiful comes is from the inside.

After three years, I realised that the real issue is not about the scars on the face, the pimples, the pigmentation but that being beautiful is inside out. When you truly accept yourself and love yourself.

After clearing my debt, I didn't know what to do. I was at a loss. I then met my first coach who guided me. I am so grateful to her. I've always believed that everyone needs a coach in life. We can't see our own blindspot. Even Tiger Woods had a coach!

She told me to write down my 100 goals and dreams! What???? I didn't even have one dream, how could I have 100? The women in my family don't have big dreams.

That was the best thing to ever happen in my life, to list my 100 goals and dreams.

Every time I asked my mum what she wanted, she always said "nothing!" She saw me struggling and she never asked me for anything.

I told her the good news that I had cleared my debts. I told her that I wanted to fulfil her dreams.

She told me she wanted to perform her pilgrimage with her mum. Wow, I realized thatthat's so urgent for me because my grandma was already old at the time. I did all I could to make this happen and we were able to go together. That was the best moment in my life.

I told myself I would make this happen yearly. And I did until it was forced to stop due to the earth cleansing (Covid).

I continued to work on and upgrade myself. I was invited to speak and share my journey in the Harvard Biz Expert Forum, Harvard University. We then wrote a book together, Thought Leaders. It became an International Best Selling book too!

I came back and was featured everywhere in the news and the media and everyone was cheering and happy for me.

Well, that is everyone but my family.

The family was embarrassed and ashamed that I spoke about us and I had been beaten up and abused by a family member. I was left alone and forced to stop doing what I was doing. I was told to choose between my family or my passion which is to tell every woman to speak up and stop abuse.

The more I spoke up, the more I kept going. But also, the more I was abused. My house was even broken in to. Yet still during that moment I was so scared to call the police. Damn all those beliefs I had from my childhood. Can you believe the abuser himself called the police and said he beat me and broke into my house?

The only shelter my daughter and I had was a rental house studio apartment for the poor but at least I had a shelter despite. This was so important to me after being homeless for years.

I'd had to send my daughter to Indonesia for two years while I fixed myself so I could give her shelter! That was the lowest moment in my life to be separated from my four year old girl. Again my mum sacrificed so much and went together with her, and I was left alone.

I kept losing people I love I had the worst abandonment issue I would do anything for the people I love to stay. Writing this now, I can't stop crying. That was how low I was, allowing people to use me so that they will love me and don't leave me!

I know it all started with the childhood I had but I know I can't blame my childhood forever. That's why I choose to heal myself and work on myself!

My brother-inlaw is now a changed man.My sister, and the entire family all accepted him back and now they are happily together with four children.! Yes, people do change. Yes, you can give them a second chance but only if you work on yourself first. Focus on your energy, let go of all the pain energy and replace it with love and compassion. This is not to say that the other person wont also have to do the work. My brother-in-law went for counselling, he worked on himself and learnt to manage his anger and violence.

I forgave the man who sexually, physically and mentally abused me. The same man who abused my mum and sister too. I teach this in my program on how to heal every part of our pain and how to break the energy and cycle of abuse. I teach how to forgive ourselves first and let go of all the energy that is stuck with the pain. It is ok to be angry, it is ok to feel all the emotions. I will hold your hand and guide you, just like I did for myself.

Living in that studio apartment was the last time I was abused. I decided to stand up again and this time shifted to a bigger house and chose to restart my whole life!

I was no longer seeking help and staying in housing for the low income.

I to a place worth millions of dollars and brought my daughter and mum back. The feeling of being able to give her a home that she asked for was indescribable. She asked for a house with pool and at the age of 27 I gave it to her.

I remember my 26th Birthday, (five years ago now). I received the best gift from my daughter who was four at the time.

It was a life awakening moment when she answered my simple questions.

I asked her "You look so beautiful baby"! Who is your mother?" She pointed at me and said "YOU"! I then asked her "Who is your father?" Again she said "YOU".

Yes, I was her mother and her father, likewise for me after my dad passed away when I was only one, my mum was both my mother and father.

It is not something that I am proud of. In fact, it is something I am here to speak up about, to break this pattern of perpetual cycle of drama, abuse, victim stories that doesn't seem to end.

Stories of men beating their wives!

Stories of men leaving their wives!

Stories of men beating their daughters!

Stories of men abusing women physically, mentally & sexually!

Stories of men saying that women are good for nothing!

I am here to break that cycle! To redesign my life and not only my life but the life of many women who is reading this and feeling stuck in the same old drama!

I continued to work on myself, money is never an issue! I always get what I want and I have the best luxury lifestyle with just me and my daughter!

In 2020, last year, i was introduced to a man, who when I spoke to him I knew he is the one! He was worth waiting nine years to find.

He believes in me, my mission and want to achieve all my goals and dreams together with me!

I want my daughter to know that she doesn't have to struggle for success. You don't have to be in pain just to get what you want. I'm loving and living that life now.

Inner work is a game-changer I attracted the man I wrote down in my love list and manifested him in my life.

Today I'm happily married, we migrated to Australia, bought two properties together and have many more to come. I'm still running my online business.

I am Bellee LV, previously known as Nabella Sd. I am an online entrepreneur mentor and personal development trainer, focusing on empowerment for women. I am also a Harvard Business Expert ForumEntrepreneurship Business School Club of Harvard University Speaker and Bestselling Author.

I have been featured in CNN 14 times, listed in the Entrepreneur Herald as TOP 30 INFLUENTIAL ENTREPRENEURS OF 2021, Straits Time, Berita Harian, Tamil Murasu and Interviewed in Oli 96.8FM and Ria 89.7FM Radio Station & SPIN RADIO UK.

I have spoken at National University of Singapore, Tembusu College and Singapore Youth Conference 2018 organized by People Association Youth Management.

I have conducted many personal development workshops for women's organisations such as Casa Raudha Women's Home and Daughters of Tomorrow Organisation, Singapore Indian Development Association (SINDA), Singapore Women Prison among many others.

At 23 years old, I was a struggling single mom who was left with $10,000 in debt and a three month old baby in hand. However, after graduating from an Entrepreneurship and Business Course, I cleared my debts in 2 months using "Her 3M" a mindset, marketing and mentorship strategy.

Now, My passion is to train more ladies to be entrepreneurs via Her Mentorship Program and Training.

As a mentor and personal development trainer, I've groomed many individuals from differing backgrounds to be more positive, healthy and wealthy and to achieve money and time freedom as a business and life coach.

Currently, I'm leading a diverse group of entrepreneurs from Gen Y, single mums, housewives, working adults and business owners to help them to make a lot of money online and aspire to create unlimited passive income so they can make more money while they sleep, spend more time with their loved ones, do the things they love with their free time in her WOW Mentorship Program!

Connect with me and let's break the cycle and pattern together. You don't have to do it alone and you certainly don't have to struggle and continue the pain. Let's put a full stop to it! I did it, the women in this book did it too! And so can you!

Always know you will be Supported!

Love and light,
Bellee LV

BELLEE LV

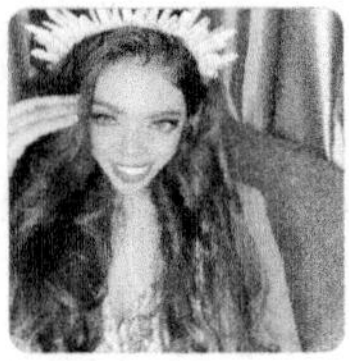

At 23-years old, Bellee LV was a struggling single mom, left with $10,000 in debt and a 3-month-old baby in hand. After graduating from an entrepreneurship business course, she cleared her debts in two months using Her 3M, Mindset, Marketing & Mentorship Strategy.

Currently, Bellee leads a diverse group of entrepreneurs from Gen Y, Single Mums, housewives, working adults, business owners to help them to make more money online and create unlimited passive income, allowing them to make more money while they sleep to spend more time with their loved ones. Her passion is to train more ladies to become entrepreneurs.

Connect with Bellee and break the cycle and pattern together. You don't have to do it alone. You don't have to struggle and continue the pain. Put a full stop to it! Bellee did it and so can you!

Website: www.belleelv.com
Facebook and Instagram: Bellee LV

12

KRISTIN STRAWDER

MY FREEDOM JOURNEY

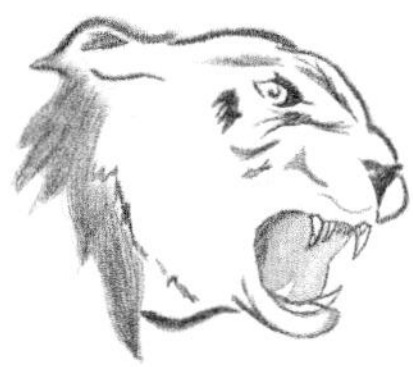

My spiritual awakening gave me the tools to heal the parts of me that kept me chained to a marriage that had passed its expiration date. It gave me my voice back, healed my emotions, and lit the way to embrace the parts of my soul that had been shattered by the years of emotional destruction happening behind closed doors. I finally woke up and saw the truth about my life and it had to change so I could fulfil the next level of my Divine mission of helping others be conscious creators of their reality and it started with acknowledging and then healing my own emotions and traumas. It was my path to freedom.

Freedom from the mind f*c*ery that domestic abuse creates. Freedom from the judgements of others, freedom to stand in my truth, embrace being a way shower and a truth seeker. Freedom to do the dark inner work to find the light in my soul again. It was hiding and simply waiting for me to be ready to embrace all of my authentic self. All the parts that kept me quiet and disconnected from myself just to survive another day in a marriage that was slowly sucking my very life force energy from my bones.

This journey to healing my life was long overdue. My soul screamed for peace daily. There was so much chaos and confusion that was preventing me from seeing the truth about my life. Even though I had made a conscious decision to thrive despite my secret circumstances, my body was flashing check engine lights at me and I couldn't ignore them anymore. I was shutting down in many ways just to function through the weekly "episodes" my life had been subjected to. I knew if I didn't heal the trauma left behind from them, that I would eventually be lost forever, I couldn't let that happen, my child needed me to be genuinely healthy, happy and thriving.

I couldn't do those things in the environment we were living in any longer. It was emotionally toxic and physically destructive and the smoke screens of deception were so thick that even I began to believe the lies said about me. In reality that was gaslighting and manipulation at its finest. All of this had to change and the change started with me.

TAKING MY OWN ADVICE

Even though I was helping other people process their own traumas as an intuitive parent coach, I was so far deep in my own survival that I didn't know where to start so I focused on what I knew best. Helping other people heal their trauma stories.

I had to start practising what I was preaching. I began to self-care when I needed it. It became a necessity to rest, breathe, dream and heal no matter what. It wasn't a luxury, it was part of my survival. I had to put my oxygen mask on first before I could help anyone else. I had to become authentic with myself and embody the journey of healing.

I began to honor my Divine mission and embrace my spiritual gifts so I could serve myself, my child, and then serve my community. I stopped pleasing people and I put up healthy boundaries. Boy, did that cause some drama. I began to speak my truth authentically no matter what it looked like or who it pleased. With time, I was able to integrate the parts of me that had disconnected while trying to silently survive a horrible situation. This process saved my life as I embraced my authentic self as the Divine showed me the path to healing.

Reconnecting to my soul essence through faith and embracing the unknown gave me the courage to rise up and advocate for myself and my tiny human. I had to give myself the same allowances that my clients received as we would work together through the layers of their trauma experienced at the actions of someone who they were supposed to feel safe and protected by.

Trauma healing can be very messy but it is also life-giving and an essential part of the freedom journey out of a DV situation.

Someone asked me recently, why didn't I just leave when all of the emotional and verbal abuse became a way of life. This was a question I had asked myself so many times throughout the years of secret terrors. I admitted that I was ashamed and afraid that the late-night threats would become my reality and I told myself that if I stayed, I could protect us better than if I left.

The shame and fear kept me quiet about the things that had been happening for most of the marriage and I was constantly masking my anxiety and fears of being exposed as a victim to something no one really wants to talk about publicly... Trauma caused by domestic violence. Each time I didn't speak my truth, I lost more and more of my soul.

Shame, terror and fear were my prison guards. My emotions were raw and being used to create situations that seemingly made me appear as the unstable party. In reality, it was the covert tactics of someone who knew exactly what they were doing to create situations to appear to be completely different to keep up with a web of deception and half-truths being told about me behind my back.

It would take me over four years and three attempts before I was successful in leaving that emotionally and physically dangerous situation. I came to terms with the fact that my reality was not going to get better and I was just prolonging the inevitable by believing the love-bombing covert attempts to keep me quiet, manipulated and shamed for wanting peace in my own home. We deserved to live in a peaceful home and our emotional and physical safety was more important than keeping up the facade that public life was the same as home life.

My yearning for peace was stronger than my need to not be painted as the villain in my very own horror story. I came to terms with the fact that I had become public enemy #1 after I took a stand against the things happening in my home that no one should have to endure. This was way more than just covert abuse but it would be a long time before I would be able to connect the dots and see the situation for what it really was.

In reality, my home was being destroyed by an emotional terrorist that was a publicly smooth-talking Casanova and a Jekyll and Hyde behind closed doors. I was hiding my light, while holding on to the hope that my home would be a safe place again despite the years of constant verbal and emotional rampaging. I was no longer willing to self sacrifice my emotional well being to someone that I needed protection from. This was not an existence of life I could thrive in long term. I wanted my child to see the joy and happiness that was possible in a safe and loving home environment.

At the same time, the mind f*c*ery and fear of the threats were so thick that I didn't seek out the protection we needed. I had been convinced that I would lose everything if I told the truth about what was happening behind closed doors. So I chose to be silent and even though some of those threats did indeed happen anyway, I am also so grateful that I do not have to live in fear anymore. I created a home of safety, peace and emotional strength so we would have a safe place to heal after where we were no longer in the constant situation of emotional turmoil. I am so grateful for this journey of healing. Taking my own advice saved me in so many ways.

The lessons learned from my healing journey as a mom, a woman, an entrepreneur, and a spiritual being having a human experience has been life changing. As an energy healer, I used my intuition and intuitive gifts to heal the emotional and energetic residual wounds of trauma which empowered my voice and my self-love journey. I am so grateful for the opportunity to live a peaceful life away from the chaos, confusion and the mind f*c*ery. It was worth the dark days to see my light shine again.

I can now see the beauty of my life-lived and I can honor my experiences as lessons learned. This has refreshed my compassion and skills to walk my Divine mission in helping others heal from their own trauma stories. I am so grateful that I am now free to speak my truth, stand in my power while continuing to heal the multi-generational impacts of DV. This allows me to hold space for myself and for others to also heal from their experiences.

The healing journey will look different to each person. Allowing the Divine to create beauty from the ashes of my life brought me supernatural comfort.

FEELING SAFE

As I began to heal from the experiences that had happened within my marriage, I had specific things that I needed to focus on to help ground me in my body and energy as I healed.

Feeling safe to express my emotions was pivotal in identifying what made me feel safe and what didn't. I would ask myself if what I was feeling (especially if I felt unsafe) was a trauma response or a healthy emotional response to the situation. This helped me recalibrate my emotions. I had to learn how to listen to my emotions and body responses again, I had shut them down to survive.

It took me a long time to feel safe in my body, my mind and in my emotions again. When I feel triggered now, I slow my breathing, ground my energy, and reach deep into my heart space while anchoring into my inner sense of safety. I refer to it in my healing work as "felt-safety."

I ask myself daily if I feel safe in my spirit, mind, body and soul.

Do I feel safe in my home and within my family?

Do I feel safe in expressing my emotions about parenting, relationships, energetic space, and is my inner child feeling cared for and heard?

Doing daily self check-ins gave me the space to stand in my power to decide what I focused on in the varied stages of my healing journey. It has been empowering. I fell in love with myself and found out what I was really made of through this time in my life.

MY TEDX TALK HELPED ME HEAL AND HAVE A VOICE AGAIN

In my TEDx talk, "Giving Your Inner Child Permission to Heal" and even in my chapter of Intuitive: Knowing Her Truth, (different last name) I talk about how trauma doesn't randomly pick someone and say today it's your turn to experience being traumatized.

No one is immune to it and every human has experienced some form of it in some way or another throughout their lifetime. For some it was from their childhood, others it was as a young adult but how we choose to heal from it is how we thrive despite experiencing horrible things.

"By looking at trauma through a different lens, it creates space for you to heal your own childhood trauma and gives you empathy for others who may be wearing their own trauma like an unspoken badge of courage."

What is your unspoken badge of courage?

Being a soul that has experienced DV is an unspoken badge of courage. It is traumatic to feel helpless to make it stop, frozen in time, wanting to fight back but don't, can't or do and it is twisted to make it look like you are the aggressor when in reality you're responding to being terrorized and emotionally beaten down.

Women like #GabbyPetito who silently took it for too long and then began to fight back are easily labelled emotionally unstable when in reality they took it for too long. Unfortunately, it happens all the time and Gabby paid the ultimate sacrifice for it with her life.

SOME DAILY PRACTICES TO CONTINUE TO HEAL THE TRAUMA

My day starts with:

Grounding my energy within my body

Prayer

Meditation

Speaking affirmations over my life, my family and my future

What are your daily practices to continue your healing process?

I try to talk to myself like I do a dog. "Hey beautiful, how are you doing today? Aren't you just a sweet thing, all smiles and always ready to cuddle on the couch. You're so happy and I love you."

All kidding aside. I attempt to be more gentle with myself whenever the inner mean girl kicks up some dust. I remind myself that healing takes time and with that comes layers of healing needed to counteract the epigenetic impacts of DV. I am proud of myself for making it this far in life.

HEALING THE ENERGETIC WOUNDS

Becoming a conscious creator of my reality took time and I had to unpack all the things that had a hold of me in my spirit, mind, body and soul. One of the areas that has helped me so much in my healing journey was using essential oils to support my emotions and the grieving process. My ability to see how there is an energetic component to the healing process was amplified. I gave myself permission to use my energy healing skills that had been laying dormant for many years to help me see where the energetic wounds were still hiding.

I set out on a journey to sever the energetic ties and heal the energetic wounds from living in silence. DV changes the neural pathways in the brain which you pass on to your children if not healed. It does the same to your children. Trauma impacts are generational. It also induces dis-ease energetically within the body over time and leaves chemical markers on your DNA genes which in turn alters how the genes are expressed.

Clearing the energetic muscle memory of trauma in the body helps tremendously with calming the stress responses. Your body keeps the score of how much trauma you experience over time.

Severing ties with the energetic vampires in my life helped a lot too. They came in a variety of different models and designs and all of them created more chaos and harm in my life until I no longer gave them access to my life.

Healing energetically will come in layers and seasons of time. Setting the intention to let it unfold gently will serve your highest and best interest.

ANOTHER WAY TO HEAL

Most recently, I have come to embrace my writing as a way to process and heal the deeper layers left to be discovered. The story of Gabby

Petito unfolding brought up more emotions for me to work through as I saw parts of me in her. From the outside looking in, it was a matter of time before something tragic occurred in that situation. Unfortunately, the wilderness became her final witness to her secret struggles.

This poem flowed from my soul the morning after Gabby's remains were discovered. The first time I saw any form of coverage from her case my spirit screamed "she's gone" days before she was even discovered. I tried to ignore what I knew to be true, the footage triggered me as I saw myself in Gabby in many ways. I was familiar with her energy and emotions during her encounter in Moab, making it hard to watch. I could have easily walked in her shoes. Her sorrow and fear were visible to me and I knew it was much more than what she was willing to admit.

I wish I had known her personally and maybe I could have shared my story with her and invited her to have a safe place to start her healing journey before it was too late.

INTO THE WILDERNESS

The silence is deafening,
The cries are silent,
The wilderness hides my screams and pleas.

My soul has been taken,
My comforts have been stripped away,
My spirit has been beaten with no marks to prove.

Triangulation.
Manipulation.
Contemplation.

Will someone hear my tormented cries?

Will someone see the signs?
Will someone help me even when I deny?

My truth is suppressed by my reactions,
My truth is silenced by what I am becoming,
My truth is screaming for me to hear my own pleas.

This won't get better,
This wilderness is here to consume me,
This darkness will blanket me as I give my last breath.

My essence is lost and broken,
My essence is morphing to survive,
My essence craves for peace.

Just give me peace!

I am separated.
I am silenced.
I am sad.

I pretend, pretend, pretend...to be okay.

I thought I was going to get a glimpse of heaven in the wilderness,
A journey through hell is what I received instead.
The wilderness was my promised land, that I barely got to see.

Empty promises of paradise to see,
Empty promises of how life will be,
Empty promises because of my need to flee.

Smokescreens and mirrors,
Secret lies to be seen,
Secretly begging for someone to see my silent screams.

So many miles, it never stops.
So many lies, it never stops.
So many calculated scenes, it never stops.

The charm.
The charisma.
The chase.

The thrill of freedom,
The thrill of fun,
The thrill of finding peace.

I seek peace.
I need peace.
I crave peace.

I wandered to the wilderness seeking peace,
I wandered through the wilderness seeking peace,
I wandered by the waters of the wilderness seeking peace.

It was never supposed to be this way.
It was never supposed to look this way.
It was never supposed to end this way.

I thought I could survive in the wilderness,
I thought I could thrive in the wilderness,
I thought I could just be enough in the wilderness.

My youth was fleeting.
My voice was bleating.
My heart was beating.

I tried to be enough, though I was already enough.
I tried to be worthy, though I was already worthy.
I tried to be authentic, though I was hiding in plain sight.

Sadly...

The mind f*c*ery still exists in the wilderness.
The demons still exist in the wilderness.
The lies still exist in the wilderness.

I will forever now be a part of the wilderness.
I will forever now be a part of the story of the untamed wilderness.
I will forever now be a part of the skies of the wilderness.

I will not be silenced anymore.
I will not be held back from speaking my truth anymore.
I will not be invisible anymore.

My voice will be heard.
My story will be heard.
My cries will be heard.

I AM NOW HEARD!

I gained my voice.
I gained my truth.
I gained my Freedom...in the wilderness.

I am so honored that this tribute to Gabby flowed from my soul. As my life has healed, I have given myself permission to express myself in ways that are vulnerable and raw at times. I now encourage you to embrace your healing journey to the fullest as well.

Sending you love, light and protection,
Kristin F. Strawder

KRISTIN STRAWDER

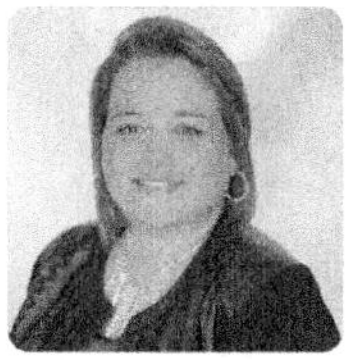

Kristin Strawder's passion is to empower women to embrace their Divine mission by embodying their spiritual gifts. As Kristin emerged from the darkest days of her own healing journey, she returned with a greater understanding of herself, and her own Divine mission.

Kristin guides moms on a path of self-transformation by honoring their experiences and lighting the way for them to implement and integrate their own feminine magic while healing their inner child.

Kristin is a momma to a spirited special needs toddler, Intuitive Energy Healer, International Best Selling Author, TBRI Practitioner, EFT Guide, Speaker, Trauma Trainer, Mompreneur, and TEDx Speaker.

Kristin serves her Healing Home Coaching online community with a free Facebook group called, The Emotional Healing Collective where all things Peaceful Parenting, Energy Medicine, Trauma Healing, Mompreneurship, Inner Child work and Essential Oils are embraced and welcomed. Kristin offers 1:1 coaching and energy shifting sessions, Live group coaching and self paced programs.

Connect with Kristin

Website: https://bit.ly/HealingHomeCoaching
Facebook Group: https://bit.ly/HealingCollective
YouTube Channel: http://bit.ly/YTHealingHome

13
BRIGID HOLDER
SPEAK UP

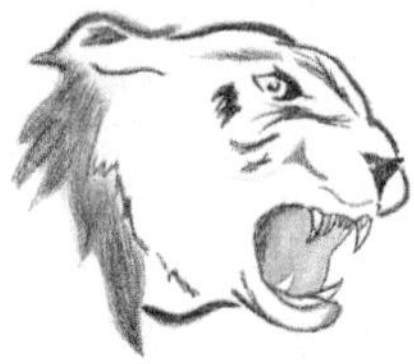

"When we speak, we are afraid our words will not be heard or welcomed. But when we are silent, we are still afraid. So, it is better to speak." Audre Lorde

The bags were packed and stood on the outside porch. They looked odd and unstable in the dim porchlight shadows. It was around 11 pm and I had gotten out of bed to use the bathroom. When I saw the precarious stack of my Father's belongings I stopped dead. Completely forgetting about the bathroom, I ran to my Dad and begged him not to leave. My Mum sat crying in the lounge room, looking afraid. I was nine years old.

At the time, I took my Mum's expression as fear of my Dad leaving her alone, but I Intuitively knew then and now that she was afraid for her safety, and with good reason. I regretted my naive misinterpretation of her expression for many years.

Of course, Dad came back. Again, and again. And at least that one time, I'm the one who begged him to stay. Was I the reason my mother went on to suffer all those additional years of abuse? Did she endure it because of me?

I struggled with the guilt and shame about that night when my childhood was ripped away from me like cheap carpet. Going forward I would have to deal with all my broken pieces as I stumbled toward young adulthood.

Was it my fault, at least partly because of that night, that someone I loved continued to hurt another person I loved? Questions like these piled up like those mismatched pieces of luggage—a heavy stack of questions I carried with me well into my late thirties.

How could I possibly meet the shame and anger building inside me? How could I avoid my growing fear of relationships and the intrinsic fear of suffering more abuse?

My mind chose the freeze method. As in when you're in harm's way, you either fight, flight, or freeze. Freezing was natural and familiar because it's how I reacted as a small child. I froze in my bed in the dark when I heard frightening sounds from across the hall.

Except sometimes I didn't freeze. Sometimes I wanted to fight back. I remember bracing myself and entering into the hall, banging on their door and yelling, "Stop it, Dad!" or "Leave her alone!". Always the same response came from inside their bedroom, "Fuck Off!"

"Fuck off, fuck off, fuck off", the two words I frequently heard over the following years that led me to drink and smoke cigarettes too young. All a crazy attempt at seeking attention from him and at the same time strengthening my defiance against him. The control did not stop just with Mum; it was with me also. And although I do not speak for them, most likely with my siblings too.

I was scared, but I continued to speak up. It's all I could do, so I did it. Sometimes the words changed; "If you are going to shoot her, you have to shoot me too!". I was 11 years old.

FORGIVENESS

> "The practice of forgiveness is our most important contribution to the healing of the world" Marianne Williamson.

I could write an entire book on all the awful things I have witnessed. Instead, I'll leave it to your imagination. I'd rather spend my words talking about how we can change society and why it's important to rally together. To share our stories. To stop normalising violence against women.

It would be easy for me to hold a grudge against and be hostile toward my Father. I've decided drinking from that poisonous, resentful cup only makes me physically sick and does nothing but fuel the perpetrator. I had to forgive him for me.

I've learned an important truth in life- that either you can become a product of your upbringing, or you can break the cycle when you question everything. You question your experiences, your perspective, look at it all with fresh eyes. With my Father, he didn't ask those questions but only dissolved into the violent cycle he existed within. And that's not an excuse for him, but now I know he's a product of his upbringing.

Violence is all my Father knew. It was heavy in the atmosphere in his environment and in his history; he didn't choose it. I could not control his behaviour back then, nor the behaviour of any other human being today. Once this dawned on me, I forgave him and let go.

There is a certain self-preservation and justice in forgiving someone and not having them as a part of your life anymore. Finding forgiveness allowed me to see more of who I am too, and I consider that a gift.

WHERE ARE WE NOW?

> "Education is the most powerful weapon which you can use to change the world." Nelson Mandela

---

Statistics tell us in most western countries, it takes a woman in a domestic abuse situation somewhere between seven to nine attempts before she leaves for good.

It's gotten worse since I helped my Mum tell Dad to leave the family home the night before exams. I was 17 years old.

At the time of writing this, statistics show astronomical increases in the number of calls to support services worldwide. Either the abuse has gotten worse, or more women are seeking help. Either way, it's appalling to know how much violence against women exists in our world. I am 49 years old.

At least once a month, there is a tragic news story about a woman, and sometimes her children, being murdered at the hands of their lover/ partner/ husband. I remember exactly what I was doing the day Hannah Clarke and her children were killed by her abusive, estranged husband. That was the final universal message for me to get this book out in the world: Hannah's death, the violent, senseless deaths of many women. We must never forget them.

I know it's a helpless feeling, not knowing what to do. But I have some ideas for moving towards elimination.

ELIMINATION

> "Overcoming abuse doesn't just happen; it takes positive steps every day. Let today be the day you start to move forward."
> Assunta Harris

I wish I believed it possible to eliminate domestic abuse entirely, but I don't; I'm a realist. Many women suffer behind closed doors, sweep their tears under rugs, hide bruises in makeup.

I believe strongly that we can work towards decreasing the abuse statistics, and here's how I see it.

• Educating our teenagers

• On healthy relationships, not just sex education. If the children don't have great role models at home, they need to learn how a good relationship looks and functions.

• On red flags, I recommend that all teens read the book 'Be Kind No Excuses' by Rie Pearson. Please give this book to your kids.

• Talk to them about their identities in relationships. Teach them about respect vs control. Have a dialogue about how both appear.

• System Upgrades

• The systems are far too supportive of the perpetrators' rights—hold them accountable for their actions and stop victim-blaming.

• Change the narrative around shame and judgement. Support victims thrown into dangerous situations and understand it's not their fault or choice.

• Talk about it (especially victims)

• Share your experience and how you found your freedom.

• Model what is possible for those without a voice or not yet strong enough to leave.

• Share in books, social media, letters if you will!

• Talk, talk, talk – get on podcasts, radio, tv media outlets to spread the word about books like this one and stories written by women who experienced abuse in any form.

SHED LIGHT ON SHAME

> "Shame should be reserved for the things we choose to do, not the circumstances that life puts on us" Ann Patchett.

Therein lies my main, most important message to all women; SPEAK UP!

• If you are in an abusive relationship – speak up!

• If you have been and you got out, speak up!

• If you suspect a friend is in an abusive relationship, speak up!

• If you can share your challenges and your wins, speak up!

• If you feel vulnerable, speak up!

• If something feels not quite right – speak up!

Leaving may be hard; it may be absolutely awful, but please do not stay for the children. If nothing else seems actionable, at least please speak up for your children - and for the generations behind them.

Thank you for being brave enough to be here, to bear witness to the very ugly, very real struggles of some of the strongest women alive. They are the lucky ones.

BRIGID HOLDER

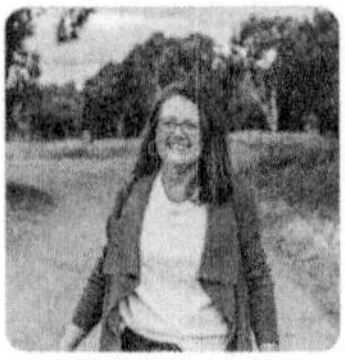

Brigid Holder is a USA Today best-selling author, multiple times best-selling amazon author and publisher, professional businesswoman and founder of The Art of Grace Publishing House. Before launching her publishing house, Brigid's many roles, both personal and professional, led her to pursue a path of personal development. A wife and mother to two teenage boys, she also helms the traditional family business as the Company Director.

Brigid started writing again in 2018 as a cathartic release. Delving deeper into her writing journey, she started to reap the benefits of publishing her own stories and became inspired to help other women do the same. The Art of Grace Publishing House, named after Brigid's beloved grandparents, serves as a safe space for women to share their stories, express themselves and collaborate to magnify their voices. Publishing both solo and multi author books Brigid nourishes her clients with her mothering ways whilst mentoring them through practical steps to become more visible.

If you are ready to share your story, you can connect with Brigid here:
www. brigidholder.com
Follow her on FB www.facebook.com/BrigidAuthorPublisher

14

ROSAANA CATALÁN

A STITCH IN TIME - SAVES 9

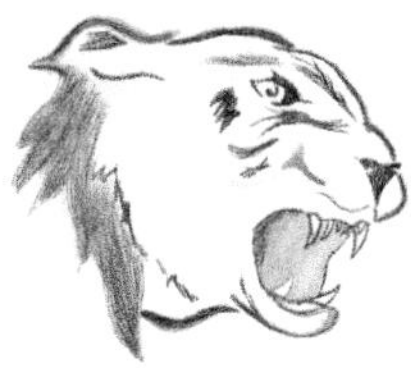

Sometimes is not enough to understand

We must believe too

Although at times we put our faith in the wrong people

And when that occurs

The only thing we can do is to understand

To believe again

And once again the mystery begins

— THE COOK OF CASTAMAR

I know what it is to suffer, to be stuck in truly paralysing ways, to go through periods of deep depression, to deal with the ongoing emotional fall out of childhood abuse; to go through a dire financial situation and turbulent times in my marriage, and to go through health issues that took a toll on me.

The point is that I have gone 'through', and I know you can too, suffering is not natural.

Suffering, whether it's happening to you, or you are in the presence of it, filters our perception of the world around us. Suffering interrupts our ability to focus our intelligence. Suffering needs to be exorcised.

If the idea of exorcising suffering appeals to you, then you know more than you think you know.

We are spirit beings, here to master our experiences of 'being human'. As such we have sovereignty over the role those experiences play in our psyche.

Mother came home from work and went to the refrigerator to find ham. My 10 years old sister had eaten the ham. She looked for my sister, found her, after shoving her face in the refrigerator, to show me her wrongdoing, she lit the gas stove and put her hands over the live fire. I still hear her screams - and the smell......

Suffering is a real thing, an emotional entity that takes our life as its own. The more we struggle, the more we feed it. Our lifeforce cannot serve two masters. My choices serve to give life to it, or to my potentially ever-emerging sense of self. And suffering ain't my choice!!!!

Although we cannot go back and change what happened. We can start again. We can reconnect to the earth that planted its fowl seed in us, pull the weed out, restore the land to balance and plant new seeds. The catch is that if suffering is all we have known, the choice we may choose to make next will yield the same crop.

Our bodies, like the land, are a gift. The gift is within. For example, when we fall and break our arm, we can go to the doctor and get an x-ray. The course of action is to bind the arm, healing occurs. The bones knit together, so why not our psyche.

Our psyche has the same healing ability as our bones do. Like our bones, our psyche needs binding, and in turn, healing occurs.

To understand anything, we become part of that which we seek to understand. To understand our potential, we are to measure our capabilities and capacities for the experiences we seek. The question for me is, how much do we understand of free will? Love? Giving and receiving care? And our power to avoid angst?

Change is natural and all around, not to change is not, self-education is the key. In-formation provides the opportunity for personal growth. Growth is natural, change is natural, change and growth are all around in nature, and we are part of nature. For us not to grow requires effort, and it is this effort that we unwittingly are applying, that opens the door to suffering. The right in-formation is key.

Once we have the right in-formation, we can give ourselves permission to live to our full potential to recreate what defines us as human beings.

Warning! Effort does not guarantee results, recreate what defines us is perfect. Perfection does not mean the absence of the negative in our lives. Negative and positive experiences are ever-present. The difference is that we can develop the ability to live with the tension of two opposing forces, existing in the same space, without folding to either.

We need to question our beliefs, how to work with them, and create them where necessary. Our knowledge of ourselves is informed by where we stand, about what we believe. The truth is that we are immaculate conceivers, this includes how we experience our world, what we look for, and where we look. However, we will only find what we believe.

Our beliefs are our emotional perspectives. Beliefs are the essential mechanisation for the process that myths and legends use to make up our internal worlds, to populate our psyche. But also as children we come armed and ready, born with natural capacities for empathy, vulnerability, curiosity, and discernment of what is the truth.

What we believe, rather our beliefs are part of our emotional DNA, working with our personal beliefs we need to be aware of them. To know what we believe is to know what the world around us looks like, it's all there, if we know how to look. We are each other's mirrors.

We have all we need, right now, we are perfect and complete to achieve what we create. Creating our experiences moment by moment, to re-educate ourselves. To look in the mirror and redefine what we see on our own terms.

"The whole purpose of education is to turn mirrors into windows" –

— SYDNEY J. HARRIS

Even today, with all that we know and understand, how to care for ourselves is a secret. WE are the best-kept secret ever told. We are living, consciously changing with every breath. Care is to come from the heart if we are to live to our potential.

Care has the power to change. To change takes timely courage. We can only change in the moment. To change a space, we are to connect to that space. To change an experience we are to connect to the experience. This is where our gifts from the heart come to work.

Empathy is the artform that transcends beliefs and creates something new. Creating new means, new to us, not from memory. To create new is to travel uncharted territories of potential. In the process of creating we face many uncertainties, it is what it is. If we then go back to gain certainty we will re-create what was already there rather than create a new consciousness.

Our conscious self is informed through empathy. Empathy with ourselves and for ourselves first. Empathy experienced through the heart, affords the awareness of the deeper spiritual union, eradicates fatigue, prevents burnout and ends loneliness.

The binding of our broken mind begins in the body, the body doesn't lie. The body doesn't lie. The body is the storehouse of beliefs. Whatever the body holds, that does not serve a renewed belief, leaves the body. With a new sense of self comes a matching body. The closer to love we theme ourselves, the greater reflections of love we will embody. It's never too late, whilst we take a breath we have the capacity to experience. Whilst we can take a breath we can change.

A stitch in time - saves 9. To withstand the force of nature and focus it for change takes effort. When I attended catholic school we had to wear stockings. I was only given one pair and had to make them last. When my stockings got a hole in them, it only took one stitch to prevent it from running. If the holes were left unattended, and the stocking ran, it would take many more stitches to mend them.

The effort of mending is called discipline. I remember when I first realised 'how to mend my soul', I wrote it on a piece of paper. I carried this piece of paper on my person for over 12 months. I practised it as a response to the 'moment' over and over again until it became my first nature. Four steps that go from looking at a mirror, and seeing what is there, to looking through the mirror to see what could be seen there. This required that I exercise my free will, and void angst.

Free will is an interesting concept. The foundation to my identity is forged in angst. Mother's foundation was forged in angst of a different kind. Her foundation was forged during the war in Spain. During the time of Franco. As a child of eight, her task was to assist the family to survive. The eldest of four daughters, she worked 12 hours a day. Part of her day was spent on the minefields. I don't choose to imagine what she was exposed to, needless to say, I lived with who she became because of it. How is that for a child, free will?

What is free will? It was not my will to be a part of the torture my sister experienced. It was not my choice to be tortured by a tortured soul. It was not my mother's choice to live in the midst of hunger, war and death. What is free will?

We are told by society that we have a choice. I ask how someone actually chooses to be treated badly at any time. As an adult, I now understand that I have choices, and the key is within me.

When I first discovered the four steps to the mantra, I was surprised to observe how few times I applied the discipline as my first choice. To realise that I was waiting for some kind of trigger, like the alarm clock telling me to get up, so that I could do what I already knew was the right thing to do. I found that if I was to follow the wisdom I had discovered I had to find a new way of thinking about discipline. It meant that I had to practice the discipline without being prompted.

I can't tell you the number of times that the only time I remembered to practise the mantra, was when I found the scraps of paper through all my clothes. You see, I had it in my pocket and didn't remove it before putting my clothes in the washing machine. It was only when I removed the clothes, I would find all these bits of paper, I would ask myself, "What's this?" I would then remember, and do the discipline then. I would rewrite it and go through the process again.

Sometimes the paper would fall out of my pocket as I pulled something else out. Or if I kept it in my wallet, it hid in the darkest part of the slit, not to be seen again until I was looking for that elusive $20 bill. In fact, that is how I began to trick myself into reading the mantra, by putting the note in places that I would find it, like the area where my driver's licence sat.

Call the experience Catharsis

Connect with your breath

Look up

Say thank you

This mantra began as words simply disconnected. After a while, they began to open parts of my mind that I needed. In order to emotionally progress through my horror-filled story and its familiar trappings of cycles of bad behaviour, bad relationships and bad choices. The Mantra was the key I was to use to interrupt feeding the monster of my habitual existence.

The Mantra afforded me a new way of thinking for answers that did not depend on the absence of my story. But from the resilience to navigate and redirect the tensions between my past that is present and the present to my future.

The greatest discovery that is ever present is that there is hope. It is time now to share this knowledge to be yours, to 'roar' with the sense of hope. I hope you can hear me. You deserve to be free too.

ROSAANA CATALÁN

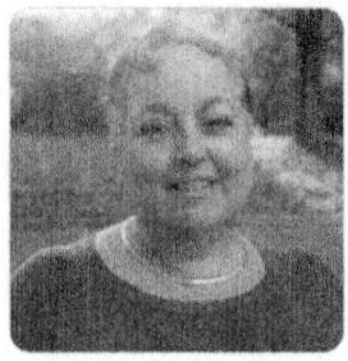

Victims advocate—everyday an idea of more.

Rosaana is a pioneer in the field of Clinical Hypnotherapy supporting women's rights to change and rise from the ashes of domestic abuse and neglect. She shares her stories, so that we may know we are not alone. Just as a broken arm heals well with the right support, so does the heart.

Rosaana, is a bi-lingual wordsmith, who for 35 years, working from the heart, guided by insight and great skills, with a wholistic approach, supports women live with self-governance, change circumstances and experience personal growth. She is a guest lecturer at Canberra University Department of Psychology; a qualified personal life coach, life's skill trainer and Pastoral Carer, with a deep understanding of what spirituality means for change.

Rosaana lives in Canberra with her husband and three adult children. She loves a good audiobook, music, rainy days to lounge around and spending time with her animals.

Email: catalanrosaana@gmail.com
Facebook: Rosaana Catalán

15

JOHANNE HOLMAN

SHE SPARKLES

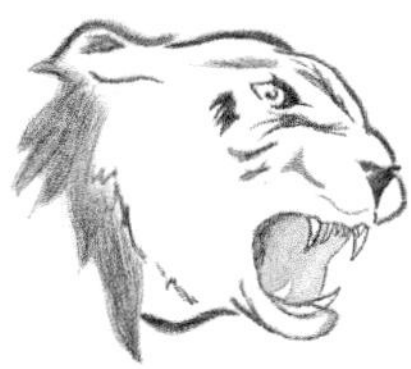

TAKE BACK YOUR POWER

RECLAIM YOUR LIFE AND RE-FIND YOUR SPARKLE

My Darling, I can only pray that you're not here reading this book, because it's you that is experiencing domestic abuse, but if it is my heart goes out to you and I want you to know we're here for YOU.

I appreciate that you may be feeling extremely empty, lost, alone, sad, frightened and confused, and it honestly breaks my heart to know this, but I can only hope that each and every one of these stories in this beautiful book, together with my platform 'She Sparkles' will help to...

COMFORT YOU to let you know you're not alone.

INSPIRE YOU to acknowledge and act on the red flags before it's too late.

EMPOWER YOU to know that there is a more beautiful life ahead.

Please be sure to take your time My Lovely, and maybe grab yourself a cup of tea, but please do read through right to the end of this chapter, to find out how you, your situation, your pain and suffering, may well now help change the world... I can't wait to see you there!

'SHE SPARKLES', HERE TO COMFORT YOU...

Feeling scared? We're here for you...

Domestic abuse is such a cruel, progressive painful thing to have to endure and the most heart-breaking reality is, there are still so many beautiful souls out there, that are totally unaware that the 'normal' that they have been living with and experiencing each and every day, is actually abuse, and I can only hope and pray that the person I am talking about here, is not you.

Too often because of our kind hearts, it can be so easy to choose to accept and excuse their poor behaviour and put it down to them having a bad day, working too hard, they've had too much to drink, they're 'frustrated', stressed, pressured, it's their childhood traumas, we literally give them every excuse under the sun, hoping to re-find that adoring loving person that we very first met.

For somebody to behave badly is one thing, we're all only human after all, but for somebody to purposely choose to behave cruelly is another, and I know the sad reality is, it won't be them trawling the internet to find out what has happened, or to see how they can change, I know My Lovely that that will be you.

I sadly don't yet know where you are on your journey but do want you to know I am here for you. Leaving an abusive relationship can be one of the hardest things that anyone can ever have to do, especially when so much of your life will have become so intrinsically entangled and entwined with theirs, your family, your home, your friends, maybe even your business. I feel for you.

Wherever you are on your journey, I am here for you, we are all here for you, and whilst I fear by the pure fact that you're reading this book, you may have already given up so much of yourself to be with them. It's my mission, whilst I rewrite my chapter, to help you rewrite yours, which is why I am so truly glad and grateful to have had you find us.

It's so easy to often ignore and suppress our emotions, and feelings, but the truth is they never lie. Our minds can play such tricks on us, leading us into these situations, believing that it's all we deserve, we're not worthy enough to have anything more or different, but I want you to know that this is absolutely not true. You've just been spending too much of your time focusing on them My Lovely, and it's time to bring the focus right back to you.

'SHE SPARKLES', HERE TO INSPIRE YOU...

If I was to ask you today... 'How are you feeling, like really feeling?', what would you say?

Would you say happy or sad?

Feeling loved or lost?

Safe or afraid?

Heard or ignored?

Supported or pushed?

Full of life or completely empty?

Comforted or alone?

Clear of thought or totally confused?

Sadly, I think I can anticipate the answer to the majority of these questions, and that heart-breakingly, you're here because you're still searching for the answers, support, understanding, and the love that you so rightly want and deserve.

You may well be feeling 'numb' right now, numb of both thought and emotion, and if you are, it's important to know My Lovely, that the only way you're going to get to heal is to pull away and to put every last bit of your precious energy moving forward, into YOU.

Wherever you are on your journey, I want to take a moment to celebrate you. I know you may well be hurting right now and feeling empty and worthless, but you're so much stronger than you think, and I hope that reading this, and all of the other chapters in this book, that it will encourage you to switch the focus away from them, and put the spotlight back on you, to start living the life you were meant to live, out fully in the light and no longer in their shadows.

If you've been sitting there with your head in your hands saying 'I don't know who I am anymore', 'I don't know what to do', 'I'm so lost', 'I'm so broken', 'I can't do this', these are words that every single lady in this book I'm sure has cried and screamed out at some stage of her journey, and look at her now. Your life, your true life is waiting for you, so let me take your hand in my hand, and comfort you on this journey, your treasure and new life most definitely await.

Knowing just how painful and confusing this journey is, I am sure that you will have spent months and months trawling the internet, listening to YouTube video after YouTube video, reading blog after blog, viewing social media post after social media post, yet don't feel any further forward, perhaps maybe even more confused than before, you're just not finding your answers. You'll have learned way more about them than you will have about your beautiful self, and that's what I am here to help you change.

Are you ready to put yourself first? Have you had enough? Are you so distraught with where you are that you just can't carry on anymore? If the answer to any of these is 'yes', you'll have just put a little bit more of a smile back on my face too, because I'll know that you will have just made the decision to start to love, treasure and take care of you.

Being in an abusive relationship is a very confusing, lonely place to be, and I can only hope and pray that you have an amazing group of friends and family around you, supporting you every step of the way, giving you a comforting hug, all the love and support and strength that you need, and that reassuring listening ear when you're telling them the same story for the 50 millionth time because at that moment, that's what you felt the need to do to help you heal.

Unfortunately, as sad as it is, not everybody has this, as they may well purposely have been isolated from you, but they really are such a fundamental part of your healing journey. Surrounding yourself with amazing strong people will help give that extra bit of comfort and protection, and if you haven't got that, then let's start creating that for you. I like to call this my RED CIRCLE.

FEELING LOST? LET'S BRING YOU HOME...

One of the biggest things that can get stripped from you is your identity, so much of your life has become about them, leaving this massive void the minute you're on your own. It can be one of the most painful realities when you find yourself unable to answer even some of the simplest questions about yourself because you've totally lost yourself along the way, or even worse, never really even truly knew yourself in the first place.

As you may well know, it's not unusual for their 'rules' to bend, flex and change from one day to the next, in order to keep you on your toes, keep you questioning yourself, and to keep you within their power and control.

A happy healthy relationship just wouldn't be this way, a happy healthy relationship would have you feeling unconditionally loved, seen and heard, but I feel sad knowing that your reality may have left you feeling a whole lot more like this, so ask you just to take a moment to imagine how different life would be if you could turn...

Confusion, where you feel like you're living with Jekyll and Hyde, into **Clarity** because you know exactly where you are?

Scared, because they've been using your 'find my iPhone' app to monitor and control your whereabouts, into **Strong** because you no longer will be controlled?

Anxious, because they just will not leave you alone, calling and calling and calling, interrupting your day, until you have no choice but to pick up, into **Confident** because you're setting and honouring healthy boundaries?

Controlled, because they've now become your wardrobe monitor, choosing and buying everything you wear, into **Independent** because you have taken back the control?

Disrespected, because they choose to scream and shout and swear at you to get you to conform, into **Respected** knowing that you will never be treated this way again?

Dishonoured, because they have no empathy or concern for how you are feeling, you can be sobbing on the floor in front of them, to only be dismissed for what they see as more important things, into **Heard** because you've finally found yourself a healthy balanced relationship?

Worthless, because of their constant need and desire to put you down and criticise you, leaving you questioning your own self-worth, into **Powerful** because you know your worth?

Isolated, because they purposely have pulled you away from the people that matter most to you, for their own selfish wants and needs, into **Comforted** because you've now surrounded yourself by loving, whole, happy, healthy relationships?

Poor, because they've taken everything from you, physically, financially, emotionally, spiritually into **Rich** because your life has become full of purpose?

Indecisive, because they've taken control of everything around you, you no longer feel confident in making your own decisions, into **Assertive** because you now know exactly where you are going and what you are wanting to do?

Frightened, because they are constantly putting the mental and physical health and well-being of you and your family at risk, because of their rages, into **Joyful** because you never will be placing yourself in that situation again?

Threatened, because they've been threatening theirs and/or your life, in order to manipulate, coerce and control you, into **Happy** because you've found the courage to go 'no contact' and remove all the manipulation and control from your life?

Fearful, because you know you don't want to be in this situation anymore, but just can't see a way out or through, into **Empowered** because you're no longer living under their power and control?

Lost, because so much of your life has become about them, into **Found** because you now know exactly who you are, what you want, and what needs to be done to get there?

It's a cruel heartless game, but not one you can't win My Lovely, if it's freedom and happiness you're searching for, it's freedom and happiness you can have. The journey won't be easy, especially if they're not ready for you to leave, but what I can say is what you can have beyond what you can see and are experiencing today, is worth so much more. You are worth so much more.

No more trying to share your thoughts, to only have them ignored.

No more giving your heart and soul, for it only to be destroyed.

No more setting boundaries to only have then smashed to smithereens.

No more trying to fix people that have absolutely no idea they're even broken.

No more being screamed and shouted at leaving you feeling worthless.

No more being bullied to do things you don't want to do.

No more wasted tears on someone who doesn't even deserve to see your smile.

No more pretending everything is fine when you're actually hurting inside.

No more, no more, no more!

'SHE SPARKLES', HERE TO EMPOWER YOU…

Are you ready to heal those wounds, to get focused on yourself, and start giving yourself the love and attention you truly deserve? Just one little step forward today could honestly make all the difference. Your new life awaits, and I can't wait to see what that looks like.

I had no idea that my life would take such a drastic change in direction but can finally now say I am truly grateful it has, because I'm here with you, and together we're changing lives.

It doesn't mean that we won't still have days when we sob our little hearts out.

It doesn't mean that we won't still have wobbles worrying about things of the future as this may well just be a part of our nature.

What it does mean is we can start to live in our truth, honouring, loving, respecting, protecting and taking care of ourselves, we can finally come home.

THE WORLD NEEDS YOU…

Domestic abuse is soul-destroying and really does need more awareness and to be taken far more seriously. There is such a stigma attached to it, with many still thinking that because there was no physical act involved, it kind of somehow makes things a little more ok. And I want you to know that what you're experiencing My Lovely, is absolutely not ok.

Abuse comes in so many different forms, psychological, physical, financial, emotional and sexual, and there isn't one less or more painful than the other, and regardless, none of them are acceptable, and it really is time for it to stop.

I chose not to tell my story, it only leaves me with a heavy heart, and if the truth be known, I am so truly grateful for every single day of my life, and what matters more to me is to now help raise awareness for Domestic Abuse, because I know there will be so many people out there, experiencing things that they really shouldn't be experiencing, having the life literally drained out of them, and I can't just sit back and let that happen and that's why I'm here for you.

As I arrive at the end of my chapter, I'm actually quite excited to realise in truth, it's really only the beginning...

WOULD YOU BE KIND ENOUGH TO HELP US TO HELP YOU...?

I really do want 'She Sparkles' to be everything you need and more, wherever you are in the world and hope that you will be able to help this happen. With your support, we can and will make a difference.

Domestic Abuse really has to be taken more seriously. It takes so much courage to leave, and a heart of steel to stay away, and even with the best legal team and court orders, sometimes, they still can't find it in themselves to leave you alone, what was domestic abuse has now become post-separation abuse, yet another cruel and painful journey.

The more we raise awareness, the more we speak out, the more we stand up to abuse, the more light we will be spreading around the world, and for that, I would be so truly grateful.

HOW CAN YOU HELP?

If you could just take a little moment more to...

- Visit www.shesparkles.co.uk by scanning to QR code in my bio.
- Click the 'help us to help you' link in the menu bar.
- Answer these three very important questions, to help us understand how you truly feel:

1. What one thing are you personally struggling with most right now?
2. What one thing (big or small) would help make your life just that little bit easier and better today?
3. What one thing would you absolutely love to see on the 'She Sparkles' platform that you feel would make all the difference for people experiencing Domestic Abuse?

It may be that you're feeling lonely and would like to be connected with somebody that truly understands how you're feeling?

It may be that you're needing a little self-love or even more some time away because you're just feeling so damn drained and exhausted?

It may be that you're struggling to find the legal and financial information you need and just don't know which way to turn?

It may be that you've left, and are so ready to start over, but have absolutely no idea where to begin?

All things, that we would of course love our platform to help you with. You matter.

AND AS A GIFT FROM ME TO YOU...

One lucky lady, of all those that choose to link through to the platform to help answer these 3 little questions will win their very own 1:1 complete Steps to Freedom program, a tailor-made hand-held step by step journey to help start to rethink and recreate their life.

Are you ready to write your next chapter? Together we can make this happen.

Sending you so much love,

Johanne xx

'SHE SPARKLES'

TAKE BACK YOUR POWER

RECLAIM YOUR LIFE AND RE-FIND YOUR SPARKLE

JOHANNE HOLMAN

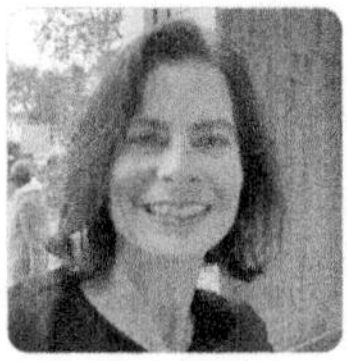

Johanne at the age of 49, courageously chose to give up every single part of the life she once knew and had been accustomed to, in order to help comfort, inspire and empower ladies experiencing Domestic Abuse.

Johanne, through her own personal journey and experiences, spent months and months trawling the internet to try to make sense of what had been going on, and soon came to realise that there was no one place for ladies to go to get the physical, financial and emotional guidance and support that they may need to help them on their healing journey.

Driven by her passion for love, kindness and positivity, Johanne is now creating an online platform 'She Sparkles' in order to help ladies all over the world, take back their power, reclaim their life and re-find their sparkle.

Website: www.shesparkles.co.uk
Instagram: @johanne.holman
Email: hello@shesparkles.co.uk

FURTHER ASSITANCE

If you or someone you know needs help... Either seek support through the women in this book or reach out to an organisation below. This only includes three countries, should you be in another please do not sit in silence—seek out the publisher and she will endeavour to look for the right avenue for you to go.

What ever your situation, it is important to know that help and support are available.

Australia
https://www.1800respect.org.au/help-and-support
1800 RESPECT = 1800 737 732

UK
https://www.nationaldahelpline.org.uk/
0808 2000 247

USA
https://www.thehotline.org/
1800 799 SAFE = 1800 799 7233

MORE FROM THE ART OF GRACE PUBLISHING HOUSE

Thank you for reading, we at The Art of Grace Publishing House love sharing womens stories. If you enjoyed this book, HEAR HER ROAR please leave us a review on Amazon or send it to us at publishing@brigidholder.com

Other Multi Author Titles published by The Art Of Grace Publishing House:

INTUITIVE – Knowing Her Truth
www.brigidholder.com/purchase-intuitive-knowing-her-truth/

INTUITIVE Speaking Her Truth
www.brigidholder.com/purchase-intuitive-speaking-her-truth/

F@#* Motherhood
www.brigidholder.com/purchase-f-motherhood/

Printed in Great Britain
by Amazon

72332224R00108